THE
FIX
DIET

ISBN 9781543926569.

Printed in the United States of America

First Printing, 2018

American Medwell
304 Genesee Street
Chittenango, New York 13037
U.S.A.
(315)687-6467

www.americanmedwell.com

A complete guide to the weight loss puzzle

THE
FIX
DIET

Four fixes for lasting weight loss

Ife Ojugbeli, MD

About the Author

Dr. Ife Ojugbeli is a board-certified internist and a certified life coach. He graduated in 1988 from the University of Lagos College of Medicine in Nigeria. After completing one year of service in the Nigerian National Youth Service Corp, he went to Trinidad and Tobago, where he worked in emergency medicine for three years. He subsequently completed his residency in internal medicine in Brooklyn, New York. He received his MBA from LeMoyne College in Syracuse, New York, and he received his CPE (Certified Physician Executive) from the Certifying Commission in Medical Management.

He is the founder and CEO of American Medwell Group and the Kudos Weight Loss Program™. He is the author of *8 Keys to Great Skin* and *5 Keys to a Healthy Lifestyle*. Dr. Ojugbeli believes that you can live a life of vitality into your 100s. During his almost 30 years of practice, including some 200,000 patient encounters in three different countries, he has seen a diversity of human problems and potential. He believes that the current epidemic of obesity and chronic diseases is a major threat to active longevity. That is why he has dedicated a significant part of his professional life to helping his patients lose weight and create health. He calls his unique approach to weight loss the FIX Diet™.

Dr. Ojugbeli enjoys running, and has completed multiple races, including the famous Boilermaker and the Empire State Marathon.

He is married and blessed with six wonderful kids.

I would like to express my sincere gratitude to my patients featured in this book for their willingness to share their results.

I am also very grateful to chef Michelle Scalzo who worked hard to put together the recipes in the book. Many thanks to Mary Beth Hinton and Victoria Lane for their assistance.

Contents

An Introductory Message from Ife Ojugbeli, MD, MBA

*I believe that the greatest gift you can give your family
and the world is a healthy you.*
—Joyce Meyer

Obesity has reached epidemic proportions in America. Statistics show that two out of three American adults are overweight or obese.[1] Some claim that as many as 97% of dieters regain all the weight they lose, some of them within three years.[2] There are more diet programs now than ever before, and there is a glut of information on how to lose weight. But the information is often conflicting, leaving the average dieter confused. From low-fat and low-calorie to low-carbohydrate and high-protein diets, how do you know what is good for you?

I must admit that, for a very long time, I applied the conventional dogma: calories in must equal calories out; that is, if you are gaining weight or not losing weight, it must be that you are consuming more calories than you are burning.

I started to challenge this notion because of my personal experience. I was rather skinny as a kid and young adult. Then in my late 20s, I started to gain weight. I watched my BMI (body mass index) go over 30, which meant that I was officially obese. Being very familiar with the dangers of obesity, I knew I had to do something.

I love to jog, so exercising was not a problem for me. I made significant changes in my diet and started to eat a "healthy balanced diet." I did lose a little bit of weight, but not as much as I expected based on the number of calories I was consuming and the amount of exercise I was doing. It was not unusual for me to run on my treadmill for an hour late at night five times a week and up to 20 miles on Sundays. I continued to carry extra weight, especially around the midsection—I often joked that the reason they call it middle age is because your age starts to show in the middle. I even ran the Empire State Marathon in 2013. My wife used to say, "You are the only person I know who runs a marathon and has a gut."

The more I researched the topic, the more I became convinced that calories are at best only half of the picture. Other factors contributing to obesity include food intolerance or sensitivity (more on that later), sugar, an out-of-balance gut, and stress. That is why I created the FIX Diet™. FIX is an acronym for Food Intolerance Xchange. The diet is based on finding out what foods you may be intolerant of and exchanging them with heathier options.

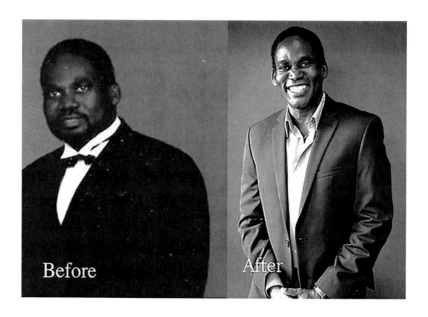

Before   After

How I Got Here

As a kid, I was skinny and loved to eat. Later, as a man in search of the good life, I traveled across the Atlantic to the warm welcome of Lady Liberty. In the US, to my palate's delight, I discovered cheese. Alas, it was no good for my waistline. Within four years my weight increased from 130 pounds to a whopping 215 pounds. On a visit to the homeland, my old neighbor, a usually polite nice lady, asked, "Who did you it?" I paused for a second and said to myself, *I hope she realizes that I went to the United States and not Papua New Guinea where cannibalism is practiced.* But I wanted to play along and have some fun. So I said, "Colonel Sanders." A long pause followed. The shock on her face suggested that she thought I might have feasted on a US military officer. I had to reassure her that I only meant some fried chicken and biscuits.

I realized then that I had to do something about my weight. What a cruel irony. I had worked so hard during my early years living in Nigeria with the hope that one day I would be able to afford any meal I desired. But when I was finally able to eat what I wanted I had to go on a diet! Unfair. But I knew better. I knew that if I was going to have the energy to enjoy playing with my kids, I would have to trim my weight. Because, like many of my patients, I have struggled to lose weight and keep it off, I know that diligence is required and that sometimes motivation wanes. That is why I became dedicated to finding a process that would deliver consistent results. The FIX Diet™ does just that.

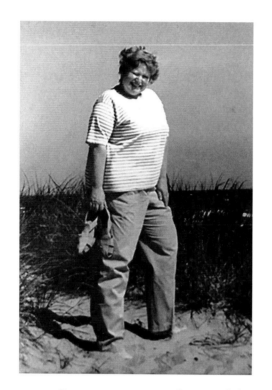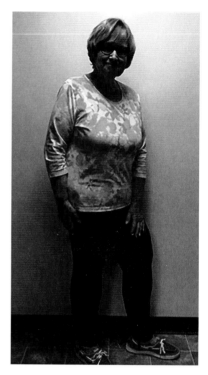

Lost 64 pounds and kept it off over 9 years.

Section 1

Understanding Obesity

Obesity is a risk factor for the development of the following diseases:

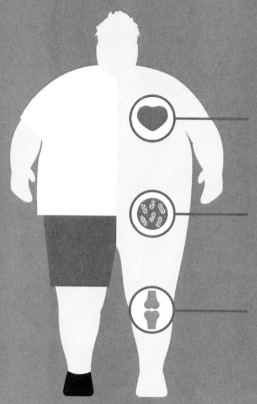

Infarction
Stroke
Hypertension
Angina pectoris
Atherosclerosis
Obesity of the heart

Diabetes
Cholecystitis
Pancreatitis
Gastritis
Violation of the endocrine
function of the pancreas
Urolithiasis disease
Obesity of the liver
Constipation

Gout
Osteoarthritis
Osteochondrosis
Spondylosis
Flat-footedness

The Consequences of Obesity

Your body is the baggage you must carry through life.
The more excess the baggage, the shorter the trip.
—Arnold H. Glasgow

L ife is a great adventure and you only get one chance at it. Therefore, it is very important to enjoy it. But to enjoy it, you must be
healthy. Unfortunately, the health of many Americans is threatened
by obesity, which is becoming a global pandemic. During the 1950s,
about 10% of the US population was classified as obese. In 2011–
2012, the Centers for Disease Control reported that approximately
35% of American adults were obese.[3]

Premature Death

Obesity-related diseases contribute to as many as 324,940 preventa-
ble deaths a year in the United States.[4] If you are a woman, having a
body mass index (BMI) of 32 or greater doubles your risk of dying
in 16 years.[5] A BMI of 40 to 45 reduces life expectancy for both men
and women by as much as 10 years.[6]

Consider these statistics: if you can't walk one-fourth of a mile in
less than six minutes, you are significantly more likely to die in the
next six years.[7] The consequences of lack of exercise and poor diet are
killing most Americans.

Chronic Diseases

Obesity increases your risk of many diseases and conditions, including

- Heart attack and heart
  diseases
- Sleep apnea
- Arthritis
- Diabetes
- Hypertension

- Chronic fatigue
- High cholesterol
- Depression

- Loss of libido
- Cancer
- Gallstones

Money Lost

Researchers have calculated how much obesity is costing individuals per year: as much as $4,879 for a woman, and $2,646 for a man. If you factor in the value of lost life and other costs associated with being obese, the annual cost for a woman sky rockets to $8,365, and for a man, $6,518.[8]

The Benefits of Losing Weight

Maintaining a healthy weight and an active lifestyle is the best thing you can do for yourself. Family studies show that only about 25% of the variation in human longevity is due to genetic factors.[9] That means that 75% may be due to lifestyle, which means that we have the ability to influence or even control how well we live and age. If we combined the benefits of modern medicine and a healthy lifestyle, we could be the healthiest people in all of history. In 1910 the average American male had a life expectancy of 48.4 years.[10] Yet today it is commonplace to see men in their 80s who are still very active.

Consider the benefits of maintaining a healthy weight and an active lifestyle:

- Better health
- Reduced risk of diabetes
- Reduced risk of heart disease
- Lower blood pressure
- Improved mood
- A better sex life
- Reduced effects of sleep apnea
- Reduced risk of joint pain and arthritis
- More energy
- Improved memory
- Improved self-confidence
- Better appearance
- More career opportunities and earning power

We Should All Be Like Ruth Colvin

Recently, I had the privilege of meeting Ruth Colvin, a fascinating woman who has become an international icon. In 1962 Ruth started Literacy Volunteers of America right here in Syracuse, New York. This organization has programs in all 50 states and in 34 developing countries. In 2006 she was awarded the Presidential Medal of

Freedom by President George W. Bush, and she is an inductee of the National Women's Hall of Fame. Ruth is now writing her 16th book, and she still works. She also exercises every day, and she plays golf and goes to the gym three times a week. Though she is 100 years old, her physical ability and vitality would be the envy of many half her age. Ruth represents what I believe is possible: that one can be active and engaged at age 100 and beyond.

Why Is It So Hard to Lose Weight?

Statistics show that two out of three American adults are overweight or obese. According to a study led by Youfa Wang, MD, PhD, of the Bloomberg School of Public Health, "If current trends continue, more than 86% of adults will be overweight or obese by 2030."[11] Still, every January 1, millions of Americans resolve to win the battle of the bulge.

The demand for solutions has given rise to a multibillion-dollar weight-loss industry. There are so many diet programs around that you can't turn on your TV or go online without finding commercials for weight-loss programs and products. A report by ABC news showed that 108 million Americans are on a diet, and the average dieter tries four different plans in a year.[12]

One problem with dieting is that, each time lose weight, you lose both fat and muscle. When you go off your diet, you regain weight. The sad fact is that you regain the fat but not the muscle, resulting in a net loss of muscle mass and a slowing of your metabolism, which makes future weight loss even harder.

Is It Just a Lack of Willpower?

My patient Jane had a lot of willpower. She had struggled most of her adult life to lose weight, trying just about every diet you could name, but to no avail. Finally, she resorted to weight-loss surgery. She did lose about 120 pounds, and she kept it off for about three years. But then the weight started to come back. Over the next two years she regained all 120 pounds and then some.

When I met her, I was struck by her tenacity in the face of significant adversities. Jane had become blind at the age of 13. Undeterred, she went on to graduate from college and complete a master's degree program. She got married and had two wonderful children. When her marriage ended in divorce, she raised her kids mostly by herself. When I met her, Jane was in her late 40s. She worked in a nearby town and took public transportation. Being totally blind, she used a stick as her guide.

On our first meeting, I walked into the exam room and introduced myself. She enthusiastically said, "I am so happy to meet you." I was impressed by her optimism and energy. This patient who could not even see me seemed so happy to meet me. I asked her how she managed to be so positive in the face of what appeared to be overwhelming challenges. She laughed and said, "Doctor, it has been much easier to be blind than to lose weight."

Easier to be blind than to lose weight? You would be hard pressed to argue that Jane had no willpower or determination.

Is It as Simple as Eating Too Many Calories?

I used to tell my patient's jokingly that if you want to lose weight, eat like a caveman—mostly vegetables and high quality protein. That was before I discovered the "caveman combo" meal offered by a famous restaurant where my daughter had her birthday celebration. I thought it would be healthy, but I was wrong: it had nearly 5,000 calories!

It is true that the average American eats way too many calories (often hidden in restaurant food). According to a study by Credit Suisse, the number of calories consumed daily by the average American rose from 3,200 in 1981 to 3,900 in 2012.[13] That is a whopping 700 extra calories a day! Within that time frame our level of physical activity did not go up. If anything, thanks to modern conveniences and technologies, we were less active than ever.

But is it as simple as X number of calories equals X amount of fat? No. Human beings are not like Bunsen burners in which a precise mixture of gas and air leads to a predictable kind of combustion. As individuals, we have unique biochemical and hormonal make-ups and circumstances. We each process calories differently, and calories themselves are not all metabolized in the same way.

I remember Jeff, a friend and colleague from my residency years. Though he ate a high-calorie, carbohydrate-rich diet, he was very skinny and his BMI was no more than 22. I'll bet most of you know somebody like that.

In contrast, many of my patients say that they don't eat much and are still gaining weight. Even patients who watch their diet and exercise regularly continue to gain weight. The conventional dogma—that if you are gaining weight or not losing weight, you must be consuming more calories than you are burning—doesn't account for such differences.

Other Factors Can Impede Weight Loss

My experience and the stories of my patients convinced me that other factors, beyond lack of willpower and eating too many calories, can interfere with attempts to lose weight, notably food intolerance, sugar, an out-of-balance gut, and stress.

Food Intolerance

Food intolerance, or food sensitivity, is a condition in which your gut does not handle certain foods well. It is not the same thing as food allergy.

How is food intolerance different from food allergy? When you have a food allergy, your body produces IgE, a type of antibody. IgE triggers the production of histamine, which in turn may cause hives, a rash, itching, and even life-threatening breathing problems. Food allergies can be detected by a blood test.

Food intolerance stimulates a much slower and milder immune reaction. With food intolerance, certain foods prompt the production of a different antibody, IgG, which is not usually detected by standard allergy tests. That is why most cases of food intolerance go undiagnosed. However, longstanding antibody production due to food intolerance can lead to chronic inflammation, an underlying factor in obesity, heart disease, stroke, dementia, arthritis, chronic fatigue, fibromyalgia, and autoimmune diseases—in short, most of the chronic diseases that plague modern humans. Chronic inflammation stresses the body, which then releases the hormones insulin and cortisol. These, especially insulin, tell the body to store fat—I once heard David Ludwig, MD, PhD (author of *Always Hungry*) refer to insulin as a fertilizer for fat cells. If you want to lose weight, you will need to reduce your levels of insulin and cortisol.

Some of the symptoms of food intolerance include:

- Bloating and gas
- Constipation or diarrhea
- Skin rashes
- Difficulty losing weight
- Brain fog
- Fatigue

The role that food intolerance plays in obesity is not addressed in mainstream medicine. It is not something I considered until I started searching for solutions to my own weight problem. I started keeping a food diary, paying close attention to how certain foods made me feel. Soon I noticed that I was eating a lot of peanuts and peanut butter and that, usually within three days of eating these foods, my skin would break out slightly and my weight would go up by about five pounds. After I eliminated peanuts from my diet, the weight came off much faster. Over a four-month period I lost 20 pounds, even while exercising less than half as much as usual. I have since tried the same approach on many of my patients with great results.

What foods cause intolerance?

So many common foods, even those considered healthy, can cause symptoms. These are the most frequent offenders:

- Gluten
- Dairy
- Soy
- Corn
- Peanuts
- Sugar and artificial sweeteners
- Eggs
- Food preservatives
- Processed foods

How is food intolerance diagnosed?

The symptoms of food intolerance overlap with those of a lot of other conditions. Because food allergy testing is usually negative, diagnosis can be tricky. There are some commercial "food sensitivity" tests available, but their reliability remains controversial. The best approach, for now at least, is to eliminate specific foods known to cause food intolerance for three to four weeks—enough time to allow your body to heal. If your symptoms improve, that is proof that you are intolerant of that food. If you are re-exposed to the food, the symptoms will most likely return.

How is food intolerance treated?

First, you identify the foods to be avoided. This can be a tedious and time-consuming process because so many common foods may be involved. I have developed a step-by-step food elimination and exchange program to ease the process.

Sugar: Is it Filling You or Killing You?

Sugar gave rise to the slave trade; now sugar has enslaved us.
—Jeff O'Connell

These days the media and policy makers devote a lot of attention to the opioid epidemic. Nevertheless, it is not the most dangerous addiction that afflicts our society today. The most dangerous addiction is **SUGAR!**

Sugar activates the same reward centers in the brain, and provokes the same cravings and withdrawal symptoms, as drugs do. Studies have shown that sugar stimulates the pleasure centers in laboratory rats more than cocaine does. When rats have the choice between sugar and cocaine, they choose sugar.

In today's world of highly processed foods, sugar is everywhere. It is in the sodas and juices we feed our kids. It is in all refined carbohydrates, such as white bread and pasta, pastries and desserts. But it is also hidden in a lot of other foods—even "diet foods." The food industry has hijacked our taste buds and our health, which is good for their bottom lines but catastrophic for our health.

The current epidemic of obesity and associated chronic diseases is directly related to the high sugar content of our foods. Here are some not-so-sweet facts:

- The average American consumes about three pounds (about 240 teaspoons) of sugar a week, or about 3,550 pounds in a lifetime.
- The American Heart Association recommends no more than the equivalent of 9.5 teaspoons of sugar a day.
- The average American adult consumes about 22 teaspoons a day.
- The average American child consumes 32 teaspoons a day.
- Added sugar alone accounts for about 500 extra calories a day—the caloric equivalent of 10 strips of bacon.[14]

When you eat sugar, your pancreas secretes the hormone insulin to process it. But when you consistently eat *too much* sugar, your pancreas produces so much insulin that your body's insulin receptors can no longer respond, a condition called insulin resistance. Excess sugar is stored as fat. It also causes inflammation, which, as mentioned above, is implicated in many chronic diseases and conditions.

An Out-of-Balance Gut

Happiness: a good bank account, a good cook and a good digestion.
—Jean-Jacques Rousseau

It turns out that your digestive health has a lot to do with your happiness—perhaps even more than a good bank account and a good cook.

The digestive system, or the gut, includes the mouth, the esophagus, the stomach, the small intestine, the large intestine, and the anus. Other parts of the system are the liver, the gallbladder, the pancreas, and the nerves, along with trillions of micro-organisms that line the gut, collectively known as the microbiome.

The gut does more than digest food. It plays a major role in immunity, appetite regulation, and even mood. We now know that more than 70% of the immune system lives in the gut.[15] The gut can protect us from infection by detoxifying and eliminating harmful substances that enter the body. Prompted by the food that we consume, the gut releases hormones that help to regulate appetite and fullness. The gut also plays an important role in mental health. About 95% of the body's serotonin, the "feel good" chemical, is made in the gut.[16] If your gut is not healthy, you may suffer anxiety, depression, and irritability.

The lining of a healthy gut is held together by what are called tight junctions. These ensure that only very small, properly digested food particles pass into the bloodstream to nourish the body. But when gut health is compromised, these tight junctions become loose and too permeable, allowing partially digested food and bacteria to enter the bloodstream, a condition called leaky gut syndrome. The immune system releases proteins called antibodies to destroy these invaders. The inflammation caused by leaky gut syndrome has been linked to most of the chronic diseases we are dealing with today, including obesity, heart disease, dementia, cancer, autoimmune diseases, arthritis, and chronic fatigue.

Leaky gut can be caused by many things, including the following:

- Excessive sugar, processed food, and gluten
- Medications, including antibiotics, acid blockers, anti-inflammatory pain killers, and steroids
- Stress, either psychological or physiological
- Environmental toxins

A healthy gut contains a diverse community of micro-organisms, with an optimal balance of good and bad bacteria. In thin people, the good bacteria predominate. Obese people seem to have a less diverse bacterial population and more bad bacteria. These bad bacteria are believed to extract excess calories from food, which is then stored as fat.

Knowledge in this area is relatively new, but growing rapidly. If you have been dieting and exercising and are still unable to lose weight, the solution may lie within.

The FIX Diet™ at a Glance

Dieting is like driving a car. When you got your learner's permit, you didn't just jump into a car and start driving. First you learned how to drive. Initially it was awkward and difficult, but with practice it soon became second nature. The problem with most diet programs is that they don't teach the skills needed to succeed. They drop a plan on your lap and you are supposed to figure out how to carry it out. Dieting successfully takes skills. I believe that mastery of dieting skills may be more important than the diet itself.

The FIX Diet™ consists of four distinct aspects, discussed in four sections below:

1. Dieting success skills:
- How to get motivated and stay motivated
- How to deal with hunger and cravings
- How to deal with stress and emotional eating and solve problems
- How to end sabotage

2. Four fixes for lasting weight loss:
- The three-phase food fix
- The gut fix
- The stress fix
- The exercise fix

3. Dealing with special challenges. This section will teach you what to do on special occasions such as during the holidays, dieting while traveling, getting past a plateau, and similar circumstances.

4. Dealing with other barriers to weight loss. Sometimes you do everything you are supposed to do and you still fail to lose weight. This may be due to undiagnosed medical problems such as hormonal imbalance or even medications.

Section 2

Dieting Success Skills

The body ACHIEVES what the mind BELIEVES

It is possible to fly without motors,
but not without knowledge and skill.
—Wilbur Wright

There are four things that could help you break free from the diet trap. These are:

1. A change in mindset. You need to change your relationship with food. Understand that food is for nourishment and not to sooth every emotion. You will learn how later.

2. Change in behavior. It goes without saying that, if you are overweight or obese, your present dieting habits and behavior are not working. To get the result you want requires a new set of habits and behavior. The good news is that, with the right skills and practice, changing your behavior is possible.

3. A plan you can follow. Just about any diet plan will work if you can stick to it. The beauty of the FIX Diet™ is that it is truly individualized. You will discover what foods are a problem for you and avoid them. You will learn good eating habits that will ensure that you eat to satisfaction.

4. Professional care. Sometimes you may need professional help. A healthcare provider with experience in weight management or a weight-loss coach can help you.

This section will teach you the four main skills you need to escape the diet trap for good:

1. How to get motivated and stay motivated
2. How to deal with hunger and cravings
3. How to deal with stress, end emotional eating, and solve problems.
4. How to end sabotage both by yourself and others.

How to Get Motivated and Stay Motivated

With the right motivation, you can do just about anything. Most dieters are usually very motivated in the beginning. Think January 1 and all the New Year's resolutions to lose weight and get in shape. Go to your local gym on January 2 any year and you won't find a parking spot. Go back three weeks later and see how empty it is. Most dieters lose their motivation too soon. This time will be different if you follow these steps:

- Define your driving desire. What's the overriding reason you want to lose weight? Is it so strong that you wouldn't compromise it? An example could be a desire to be able to play basketball with your grandchildren even at age 65. Now that is something to work for and be uncompromising about. One of the patients I worked with simply said her reason for losing over 100 pounds was because she did not want to die.
- Set goals.
- Create a plan.
- Take actions based on your plan.
- Track your activity.
- Reward success.
- Amend errors.
- Win or learn.
- Never give up.

It is important to look at weight loss as a lifelong journey. You don't want to start without a clear road map. I created the 3D Analysis™ to help you lay the groundwork for a successful weight-loss journey. The three Ds stand for **desire(s), dangers,** and **doable** analysis. The 3D Analysis™ is a series of exercises designed to help you uncover why losing weight is important to you in the first place. It will also help you anticipate vulnerable occasions and create plans to deal with them. I do not want you to skip this crucial first step. In fact, I want you to take the exercises very seriously and thoughtfully and put in place action steps, which will make all the difference between success and failure.

Desire(s)

The first thing you have to do, even before you think of your diet plan, is to think hard about why you want to lose weight. You need to uncover a reason strong enough to drive you through the challenges that are sure to come. Discovering your driving desire is different from merely setting a goal, as important as that may be. A goal is usually a logical left-brain idea. You need a strong desire to motivate you to make needed changes. Well chosen questions can provoke a powerful emotional response. This is what the 3D Analysis™ will do for you. Since your reason may not be immediately obvious, ask yourself these questions:

- A year from now, what three things, with respect to your health, will make you feel happy, content, and pleased with your progress? This question is a variation of what Dan Sullivan (founder of Strategic Coach) calls the R-factor (relationship-factor) question.
  1. _____
  2. _____
  3. _____

- Why will these things make you happy? The answer to this question will most likely reveal your true driving desire.

  _____
  _____
  _____
  _____
  _____

It is fascinating to see my patients do this exercise. It is usually the first time they are actually contemplating what will make them happy with regards to their weight-loss journey and why.

Do this now: Transfer your answers to the above on an index card that can fit in your wallet. Call it "My Reason Card." Read it every morning and every evening for no less than three months. Also read it whenever your resolve starts to weaken.

Dangers

Now that you have clearly identified your driving desire, it is time to work on the second D: the dangers. First, you anticipate the times when you are likely to succumb to temptations so that you can develop the skills you'll need get through those times unscathed. Second, you prepare to deal with such moments. Third, you plan what to do when you suffer a setback—because, even with the best intentions, most of us will have setbacks from time to time.

- What are five potential occasions when you are likely to be tempted to make the wrong food and drink choices?
    1. _____
    2. _____
    3. _____
    4. _____
    5. _____

- What are five action steps you can take to deal with these temptations?
    1. _____
    2. _____
    3. _____
    4. _____
    5. _____

These action steps are essential tools in your tool box. I recommend you take time and care to come up with the answers.

Here is my own dangers analysis. For me there are five danger times when I feel most tempted:

1. At dinner time

Action plan:
- Plan dinner ahead of time.
- Have a consistent dinner time.
- Change out of work clothes before sitting down for dinner.
- Drink a glass of water five minutes before dinner time.
- Eat slowly and spend no less than 20 minutes eating dinner.

2. At parties

Action plan:
- Have a small salad before the party. That way I am not very hungry at party time.
- Figure out what is on the menu and decide what I am going to eat at the party.
- Focus more on socializing and less on the food.

3. When vendors bring goodies to the office

Action plan:
- Bring my meals and healthy snacks to work.

4. While traveling

Action plan:
- Pack healthy snacks.
- Have fallback choices such as a healthy salad.

When under stress

Action plan:
- Become mindful of getting out of control.
- Practice deep breathing exercises.
- Have healthy options readily available.

Even with the best plans, at some point I am going to have a setback. It is important to have a come-back strategy from a setback. What will I do to get back on track after a setback?

- _____
- _____
- _____

Action plan:
- Keep a food journal.
- Plan meals at least one day ahead.
- Honor my plans including my exercise plan.

Do this now: Create your "My Fight Back Temptation Pledge."
On the reverse side of your My Reason Card, write the following:
As much as I am tempted to _____, the pleasure is only temporary, and losing weight is more important to me. Besides, if I give in, I will feel guilty, but if I resist I will feel great. I'd rather feel great than guilty.

Read this in the morning and evening and look for opportunities to practice your new skill.

Doable Analysis

> *By failing to prepare, you are preparing to fail.*
> —Benjamin Franklin

This is the stage when you get down to business. This is the time to create your plan.

What can you do to ensure success?

1. Set goals. A smart goal should be
- Specific
- Measurable
- Achievable
- Result oriented
- Time-bound

An example of a smart goal is "I want to lose 20 pounds in four months." It is specific, measurable, achievable, result-oriented, and time-bound.

1. Improve your dieting skills. Just like any other skill, you need to practice your dieting skills on a regular basis. The good news is that you will improve. When you do, dieting will seem to require less effort. Here are some additional skills that will help you.

How to Deal with Hunger and Cravings

Hunger is defined as a feeling of discomfort or weakness, coupled with the desire to eat. Inherent in the definition is the fact that hunger is caused by a lack of food. However, the desire to eat in of itself does not mean that you are hungry. It is very important to learn how to tell the difference between the two. If you have a desire for food but you are not hungry, remember that *if hunger is not the problem, food is not the answer.* But if you are truly hungry, you need to learn to eat the right types of foods, in the right amounts, at the right time, and in the right manner.

Tips for Controlling Hunger

- Follow a meal schedule. This will help you to avoid unplanned eating.
- Plan your meals at least one day in advance.
- Be prepared. Prepare or pack what you need. Know what you are going to eat before meal time and make sure you have it ready.
- Gut check. When you feel the desire to eat, take a deep breath and pay attention to how your stomach feels. Is it empty? Are you weak? Are you hungry or is the desire due to something else?
- If you are hungry and it is reasonably close to your meal time, go ahead and enjoy your meal, but eat mindfully. More on that later.
- If you are not hungry, then don't eat. Try drinking water or tea, or distract yourself with other activities. The desire will pass quickly.
- Use your My Fight Back Temptation Pledge.

- If you are getting hungry before your scheduled meal time, consider scheduling snacks in between meals.

Practice Mindful Eating

Look at the time when you sit down to eat, and take at least 20 minutes to eat your meal.

- Chew your food completely.
- Put your fork down between bites.
- Talk to your family and friends and ask about their day.
- If you are eating alone, notice something in your surroundings such as a painting and focus on it for a bit.
- Take sips of water during the meal.
- Pay attention to how you feel.
- Stop eating when you feel satisfied and not stuffed.
- Don't worry about finishing everything on your plate.
- Notice the difference between satisfaction and feeling over-full.
- Practice mindful eating at every meal.

Stay Full on Healthy Snacks

- Raw veggies
- Roasted veggies
- Fruits
- Nuts
- Boiled eggs
- Plain yogurt and berries (after your restoration month—more on that later)
- Cheese sticks (after your restoration month).

Deal with Temptations

- Get rid of all tempting foods in your fridge, pantry, and kitchen.
- Rid your office of tempting foods.

- Learn to politely decline food pushers.
- Use your My Fight Back Temptation Pledge.
- Drink water or a cup of tea.
- Distract yourself with other activities.
- Don't socialize in the kitchen.
- Shop from a grocery list.
- Don't go to the grocery store hungry
- Shop the perimeter of the grocery store and avoid the junk food aisles.
- Use smaller plates.
- Remember that if hunger is not the problem, food is not the answer.

Deal with Cravings

A craving is an overpowering desire for a certain food or foods. The foods that we commonly crave are sweets, salts, gluten, processed foods, and dairy. These same foods have been associated with leaky gut syndrome. Leaky gut has been linked to inflammation and increased risk of autoimmune diseases, arthritis, joint pains, mental fog, bloating, constipation, diarrhea, heart disease, heart attack, cancer, dementia, and more.

Even though cravings seem overpowering, they can be controlled. Experts estimate that cravings usually last only about three to five minutes. That is good to know. I'll bet you thought they lasted much longer. Here are some tips:

- Make a mindset shift.
- Would you eat your favorite candy bar if it was dipped in arsenic? My guess is no.
- Condition your mind using the pleasure-pain principle. Pain is more immediate than pleasure, which means that we focus on avoiding pain before seeking pleasure.

- Think of the food you crave and link it to the dangers it causes such as leaky gut. Picture the food in your gut, causing the gut lining to loosen and leading to leaky gut and inflammation.
- After a while, your brain will associate the food with danger, which will make it easier for you to say no.
- Remember that cravings are temporary and will soon pass. But the consequences of giving in will last much longer. Is the temporary pleasure worth the long-term pain?
- Use your My Fight Back Temptation Pledge.
- Don't have tempting foods around.
- Don't go hungry. Follow your meal schedule.
- Drink water and stay hydrated.

Try These Substitutions

- Whole fruits for sweets
- Sparkling water with berries or a slice of orange for sodas
- Roasted veggies for chips
- Almonds or dark chocolate for milk chocolate
- Frozen banana smoothie for ice cream

If you are still struggling with cravings, consider getting professional care.

How to Deal with Stress and Emotional Eating

The late Dr. Norman Vincent Pearle once said that problems constitute a sign of life. During your lifetime, you are always going to be dealing with problems. Some are small and some are large. The key is not to be afraid of problems but to face up to them when they arise.

What causes the experience of stress is not really the event. It is the interpretation we give to the event that causes us to feel stressed. The good news is that, as an adult human being, you can decide what meaning you will give to any event in your life. If somebody cuts you off on the road, you can choose to think that it was the driver's problem—or you can become enraged.

Jim Rohn once said that when it comes to dealing with life, "Don't wish for less problems, wish for more skills."

Five Steps to Mastering Stress

1. Acknowledge the problem. Don't bury your head in the sand. If you do, the problem will fester and will most likely come and bite you harder later.

2. Define the problem. A problem clearly defined is a problem half solved.

3. See the problem as it is. Don't magnify it, as many of us tend to do. Don't minimize it either. How would your logical friend see the problem?

4. Take care of the problem. It is not what happens but what you do that is more important. Action gives you a measure of control. Your options are to avoid, alter, adapt, or accept the cause of the stress. Here are some action steps for effectively dealing with problems:

- Define the desired outcome.
- Ask, what are the obstacles between you and your desired outcome?
- Ask, what strategies could you use to overcome the identified obstacles?
- Ask, what opportunities can you take right now to get the desired outcome?
- Break down the strategies into specific action steps, from complex to simple.
- Create an action plan.
- Take the first step.
- Evaluate the results.
- Adjust your actions accordingly.

5. Take care of yourself. Whenever we are under stress, we tend to abandon our needs and forget to take care of ourselves. This is an interesting paradox. The truth is that the more stress you are under, the greater your need to take care of yourself. I cannot count how many times a patient has said to me, "I couldn't eat well because I was under a lot of stress." Stress lowers your immunity. If you eat poorly, don't exercise, and don't get a good night's sleep or learn to relax, you are likely to burn out sooner rather than later. You must take better care of yourself when your stress level is high. You owe it to yourself and those who depend on you. Here are some things you can do to take care of yourself:

- Eat healthy.
- Exercise.
- Meditate.
- Listen to music.

- Call a confidant.
- Seek out comedy—laughter is the best medicine.
- Build your support system before you need it.
- Create a rejuvenation list of healthy activities.

Steps to End Emotional Eating

- Gut check. When the desire to eat strikes, take a deep breath and have a gut check. If you are not hungry, then don't eat.
- Remind yourself that the desire will pass quickly, but if you give in, the guilt will last much longer.
- Use your My Fight Back Temptation Pledge.
- Remind yourself of why you want to lose weight.
- Define the emotion causing the temptation.
- Deal with the source of the emotional discomfort.
- If you are bored, find something to do such as taking a walk, completing a chore, or calling a friend.
- If you are worried, write in a journal, call a confidant, meditate, or exercise.
- If stressed, try some of the stress management techniques discussed earlier.
- Congratulate yourself for not giving in.
- If you give in, try again the next time an opportunity presents itself.

How to Deal with Sabotage by Yourself and Others

Old habits die hard. You need to constantly monitor yourself. Your old thinking and behaviors will soon try to creep back into your routine. Be ready to recognize them and deal with them accordingly. Remember: if you practice your skills more, you will need willpower less. Self-sabotage is just an excuse for failing to prepare. Be completely honest with yourself.

Five Steps for Dealing with Sabotage

- Recognize what you are doing to defeat yourself.
- Remind yourself of how important weight loss is to you.
- Build resolve. Don't excuse yourself. Remind yourself of the benefits of losing weight. Use your My Fight Back Temptation Pledge.
- Take alternative action. Do something else rather than eat.
- Congratulate yourself if you succeed in overcoming the sabotage, or be prepared for the next time.

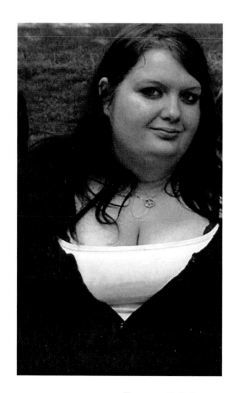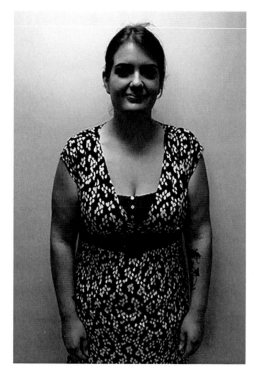

Lost 110 pounds over 3 years.

Four FIXES for Lasting Weight Loss

These are the four fixes for lasting weight loss:

- *The food fix (in three phases)*
- *The gut fix*
- *The stress fix*
- *The exercise fix*

The Three-Phase Food Fix

Phase 1: Restoration

The first phase is designed to restore your gut and heal your system from the impact of foods and a lifestyle that has been toxic to it for a long time. During this phase, you will eliminate foods that cause food intolerance and chronic inflammation. You will substitute these with alternatives that are nutrient rich and healing. You will also take additional steps including micronutrient support to heal the gut. You will learn to relax and begin a sensible exercise routine. This phase lasts 30 days. See The Restoration Phase, which begins on page 51.

Days 1 to 30

- Use the FIX Diet™ (The Food Intolerance Xchange diet). Choose from the preferred list and avoid foods in the eliminate list.
- Cut sugar, gluten, and processed foods from your diet.
- Plan your meals at least one day ahead.
- Eat mindfully; eat slowly. Take 20 minutes to eat your meal.
- Drink at least 64 ounces of water daily.
- Eat three meals and two optional snacks.
- Do not skip breakfast.
- Eat vegetables and fruits, high-quality protein, and healthy fats with every meal.
- Half of your plate should be vegetables and fruit, a quarter lean protein, and a quarter healthy fats.
- Do not eat within two hours of going to bed.
- Track your food intake.
- As much as possible, buy organic whole foods.

- Thoroughly wash produce to eliminate any pesticides and toxins.
- Eat wild-caught fish and free-range, grass-fed poultry and beef whenever possible.

Phase 2: Transition

During this phase, you will begin to re-introduce certain foods that were eliminated in the previous phase. You will monitor how you feel when exposed to the food. If you feel poorly, then you are probably intolerant of the food. You will have to avoid it for a little longer or maybe for a long time. The duration is variable depending on individual experience.

Days 31 to 60

- If you are feeling good and happy with your results from the first 30 days, then you are ready for the re-introduction phase.
- If you are not satisfied with your results, you can continue the program for the first 30 days.
- You may re-introduce the food groups avoided in the first 30 days.
- Introduce one food group at a time.
- Try the new food for three consecutive days. If it makes you feel bad, then you should avoid it for a longer period. You may retry it after about three months or you may elect to avoid it altogether.

Phase 3: Maintenance

This phase is when you have fine-tuned your program. This is how you will live for the long term. You will be eating only foods that nourish you while avoiding those that make you fat and unhealthy. You will know how to heal your gut, effectively manage your stress, and enjoy fun activities. To get the best result, it is very important to follow the recommendations as much as possible.

Day 61 and Beyond

- Transition to the Mediterranean diet.
- Modify your diet based on any identified food sensitivities.
- Avoid any foods that trigger symptoms of food intolerance.
- Continue to take fiber and supplements as outlined below.

The Gut Fix

- Increase fiber intake; take at least one fiber supplement a day.
- Make sure to get five servings or more of vegetables in a day.
- Take a high-quality probiotic.
- Take vitamin D.
- Help repair the gut with supplements such as omega-3 fatty acids and glutamine.
- Take digestive enzymes if needed.

How to Heal the Gut

There are four ways to heal the gut (the 4R principles):

1. Remove foods that are toxic to the gut such as sugar and processed foods and, for some people, gluten and dairy.
2. Replace with foods that support gut health, including whole foods and fiber. Fiber is considered a prebiotic, that is, it promotes the growth of beneficial bacteria in the gut.
3. Re-inoculate with healthy bacteria, also known as probiotics (more on probiotics below).
4. Replenish the gut with healing supplements such as omega-3 fatty acids, vitamin D, glutamine, and quercetin.

What Are Probiotics?

Friendly bacteria are vital to proper development of the immune system, to protection against microorganisms that could cause disease, and to the digestion and absorption of food and nutrients.
—National Center for Complementary and Alternative Medicine

In 2013 the Internal Scientific Association for Probiotics and Prebiotics (ISAPP), defined probiotics as "live microorganisms that, when administered in adequate amounts, confer a health benefit on the host." In other words, probiotics are the friendly bacteria, and they help to keep us healthy.

More and more people are consuming probiotics daily. However, probiotics have always been in our bodies. While being born, babies pick them up in the birth canal, unless they are born by cesarean section. Such babies seem to have a higher incidence of allergies and other health issues.[17]

We need good bacteria to crowd out bad bacteria, which has been shown to cause fat storage and obesity. Probiotics are useful in the treatment of

- obesity
- infectious diarrhea
- antibiotic-associated diarrhea
- irritable bowel syndrome
- bloating
- ulcerative colitis
- fatty liver

Probiotics also help to boost the immune system. The immune system's main job is to fight off anything that invades or threatens health. If your immune system is weak, you are likely to be overrun by disease and poor health. There is emerging evidence that probiotics can also enhance the health of the reproductive system and the oral cavity, and they even improve mood.

There are many types of probiotics. The type of probiotic you take should in part be determined by what you are trying to achieve. Here are some of the probiotics:

Bifidobacteria: There are over 30 species of Bifidobacteria, and they constitute most of the healthy bacteria in the colon. They enhance tolerance of lipids and glucose. They also crowd out the bad bacteria such as Firmicutes, and in so doing enhance weight loss. Bifidobacteria also help with irritable bowel syndrome, bloating, abdominal discomfort, and digestive disorders.

Lactobacillus: These are found in the digestive tract, and in the genitourinary system. There over 50 species. They enhance resistance to yeast infections, bacterial vaginosis, diarrhea, urinary tract infections, skin conditions such as eczema and acne, and canker sores. They are also helpful with lactose intolerance.

Saccharomyces boulardii: This is the only yeast probiotic. It is helpful for diarrhea, Clostridium difficile enteritis, and acne.

Streptococcus thermophilus: This produces the enzyme lactase. It is therefore useful for people with lactose intolerance.

Others probiotics are Enterococcus feacium and Leuconostoc.

These are some food sources of probiotics:

Kefir: Contains both bacteria and yeast. One study showed that kefir may be helpful with controlling blood sugar in diabetics. During an eight-week period, people with diabetes were given kefir milk versus conventional fermented milk. Those who got kefir had a significant reduction in their hemoglobin A1c.

Kimchi: Some studies show that kimchi may have anticancer benefits. It also helps with obesity, constipation, skin health, and overall colon health.

Yogurt: Contains Lactobacillus, Streptococcus thermophiles, and Bifidobacterium. It is helpful for gastrointestinal diseases and lactose intolerance, allergies, type 2 diabetes, and respiratory diseases.

Other food sources of probiotic include sauerkraut, tempeh, sour pickles, and aged soft cheese.

The Stress Fix

- Do deep breathing exercises daily.
- Meditate daily.
- Sleep (get between six and eight hours a night).
- Take warm baths.
- Get massages.
- Listen to music that you enjoy.
- Create your rejuvenation list and chose from there.
- Take care of the problem causing the stress. Don't bury your head in the sand.

Unmanaged Stress

> *We live well enough to have the luxury to get ourselves*
> *sick with purely social, psychological stress.*
> —Robert M. Sapolsky.

At a time in human history when we enjoy an abundance of material goods and conveniences, we are highly stressed. Compared to our great grandparents, we seemingly have it easy. We should be happy and healthy. Instead, we suffer from obesity and other chronic diseases.

Stress results when we perceive a threat or danger, whether from a bear in the woods or an unhappy boss. The so-called fight or flight response involves the sympathetic nervous system, which controls respiration, heart muscle function, and digestion, as well as the hormones adrenaline and cortisol, which cause the heart to beat faster and to increase the flow of blood. Glucose and fat come out of storage to provide energy for fast action.

A performance-boosting stress reaction could save your life if it helped you avoid a runaway tractor trailer or some other danger. However, continuing stress—over money, job security, work-life balance, conflicts with family and friends, and world events—is bad for your waistline and your overall health.

Unrelenting stress leads to persistently high levels of circulating cortisol and insulin, leading to fat storage, especially in the midsection. In addition, stress has been shown to affect food choices and eating behavior and even the distribution of fat in the body. While feeling stressed, many people crave "comfort foods" that are high in fat and sugar. Is it a cruel joke that "stressed" is "desserts" spelled backwards? Eating foods high in fat and sugar in the presence of elevated cortisol and insulin is a recipe for weight gain and obesity. It is akin to having good seeds and fertilizer. You can expect to blossom. Weight causes more stress, which leads to more weight gain—a vicious cycle.

Stress cannot be avoided completely. Just when you finished fixing the roof, the fridge goes. If you are not worrying about money, you are worrying about health or relationships or politics. The best thing to do is to become better at handling stress. If you want to lose weight and be healthy, you need a daily process for dealing with stress in your life.

I often tell my patient that when you are under stress you have two main responsibilities:

1. Take care of the problem that is causing the stress.
2. Take care of yourself. This is even more important when the problem cannot be solved right away. Unfortunately, when most people are under stress they become so focused on dealing with the problem that they ignore themselves. This is when they stop exercising because of lack of time and start making poor food choices. Before long obesity sets in, along with chronic diseases.

The Exercise Fix

- Exercise at a moderate pace for 30 minutes or longer at least five days a week.
- Do interval training at least three times a week (an alternative to the above, but if you are not used to exercising, you should consult with your health care provider first).
- Do resistance training at least twice a week.
- Stretch every day.

The Problem of Inactivity

Data from the Centers for Disease Control and Prevention indicate that the percentage of Americans aged 18 and over who meet the physical activity guidelines for both aerobic and muscle-strengthening activity is 21.7%.[18] The conveniences of modern life have contributed a great deal to sedentary lifestyles and inactivity. Many people find it hard to maintain a regular exercise routine.

The key to changing exercise habits is to make them into a ritual, just like brushing your teeth, taking a shower, or going to work. To accomplish this

1. Decide what cardio and resistance exercises you will do.
2. Decide when and how often you will do them.
3. Create space in your schedule.
4. Commit to your program.
5. Start slowly.
6. Start with something you enjoy.
7. For example: I will go for a 30-minute brisk walk three times a week and strength train twice a week.
8. Decide on the specific times that you will exercise. For example: I will go for a brisk walk from 6:00 p.m. to 6:30 p.m.

on Tuesdays, Thursdays, and Saturdays. I will strength train from 6:00 p.m. to 6:30 p.m. on Mondays and Wednesdays.

9. You must commit yourself to the schedule

Exercise prescription

The following are key elements of a good exercise prescription:

1. Frequency. The American College for Sports Medicine recommends a minimum of 150 minutes of moderate intensity exercise per week (30 minutes, five days a week) to improve health, and 200 to 300 minutes per week for long-term weight loss (40 to 60 minutes, five days a week)

2. Intensity. Use a moderate pace, such as a brisk walk—a pace at which you can still converse but not sing.

Many types of exercises

There are very many ways to meet your exercise goals. It is not necessary to belong to an athletic club to stay active. However, if you have the time and money to join one, it might give you the motivation to build regular exercise into your daily routine. You need to find an activity that you enjoy so that you can stick with it for the long haul. Remember: the older we get, the more we need to stay active. Here are some of the activities you can participate in:

Walking—a great way to stay active. The goal is to take about 10,000 steps a day. You don't have to do this all at once. You can spread it throughout the day if you wish. There are many tracking devices available today.

Aerobics classes	Weight training
Jogging	Golf (you should carry your
Running	clubs and walk rather
Swimming	than use the cart)

Tennis	Rowing
Basketball	Squash
Badminton	StairMaster
Bicycling	Wii Fit
Elliptical machine	Hockey
Racquet ball	Softball
Soccer	Baseball
Cross-country skiing	Frisbie and Ultimate Frisbie
Hiking	Yoga
Rollerblading	

You can add many more to this list. What is important is that you find an activity that you enjoy and are likely to stick with. Sometimes finding a buddy to exercise with is a great idea. It makes exercise more fun and helps to hold you accountable.

Whatever you do, you should start slowly and work your way up as your endurance improves. You should strive to do at least three days of cardio workout and two days of weight or resistance training per week.

Resistance exercises

With resistance machine:

1. Leg press
2. Leg curls
3. Quadriceps extension
4. Calf raises and toe raises
5. Hip abduction and hip adduction
6. Chest press
7. Shoulder press
8. Pull downs
9. Bicep curls
10. Triceps extensions
11. Plank

Without resistance machine:

1. Squat with feet shoulder width apart
2. Hip raises with chair or ball
3. Calf raises and toe raises
4. Hip abduction and adduction
5. Wall/modified/floor push ups
6. Shoulder press with resistance bands or weights
7. Pull ups
8. Bicep curls using resistance bands/weights
9. Chair dips
10. Plank

Non-exercise-activity, or thermogenesis

Structured exercise is not the only way to burn calories. Any muscle activity leads to energy expenditure. Thermogenesis, or the production of heat in the body, happens even while we are carrying out daily activities that are not considered exercise, such as doing dishes, doing the laundry, taking the garbage out, and going to get the mail.

Tips to increase thermogenesis

Park farther out when you go to such places as the mall or the store.

Take the stairs instead of elevators.

Walk to your coworkers' offices rather than using the phone.

Do dishes and hang laundry out to dry.

Use a push mower instead of a riding mower.

Stand up several times during your work day if you have a desk job.

Walk to lunch.

Section 4

Implementation

The Restoration Phase

The FIX List™ (Food Intolerance Exchange List)

FOOD GROUP	ELIMINATE	SUBSTITUTE
Gluten containing foods	Wheat (whole wheat or white) bread Rye Barley All brans Pasta	Brown rice Quinoa Sweet potato Gluten-free oats Gluten-free pasta Legumes Lentils Nonstarchy vegetables
Dairy	Milk Buttermilk Cream Butter Cheese Yogurt Ice cream Chocolate Whey protein powder/shakes	Almond milk Coconut milk
Sugar and artificial sweeteners	White/brown sugar Sweetened drinks/juices Jam and jelly High fructose corn syrup Maple syrup Soda Diet soda Juices	Xylitol Coconut sugar Sparkling water Stevia Erythritol Raw organic honey

FOOD GROUP	ELIMINATE	SUBSTITUTE
	Fructose Splenda Agave NutraSweet Saccharin	
Nuts	Peanuts/peanut butter	Almond butter Cashew butter Pecans Pistachios
Others	Soy Eggs Corn	Avocado Coconut Chia seeds Flaxseed Lean protein

The Sugar Exchange List

FOOD GROUP	ELIMINATE	SUBSTITUTE
Drinks	Beer Fruit juices Soda Diet soda Crystal light Gatorade Champagne Sweet tea Sweetened drinks Enhanced H_2O (sweetened) Energy drinks Wine Kool-Aid	Water Sparkling water Tea Lemon-Aid Unsweetened coconut water Organic coffee Decaf coffee

FOOD GROUP	ELIMINATE	SUBSTITUTE
Dressings/sauces	Balsamic dressing Balsamic vinegar Marinara sauce (added sugar) BBQ sauce Blue cheese dressing Catalina dressing Honey mustard Peanut sauce Cocktail sauce French dressing Ranch dressing Steak sauce Thousand Island dressing Raspberry vinaigrette Teriyaki sauce Tartar sauce	Red wine vinaigrette Olive oil Avocado oil Salsa Marina sauce, unsweetened Mustard Sesame oil Tabasco Vinegar Caesar dressing Italian dressing Tomato sauce
Grains	Wheat (whole wheat or white) bread Rye Barley All brans Pasta	Brown rice Quinoa Sweet potato Gluten-free oats Gluten-free pasta Legumes Lentils Nonstarchy vegetables Black beans Wild rice Chickpeas Coconut wrap Lima beans Hummus Rice pasta

Preferred Meal Options

FOOD GROUP	PREFERRED
Vegetables	Broccoli
	Brussels sprouts
	Spinach
	Kale
	Cauliflower
	Red peppers
	Artichoke
	Garlic
	Eggplant
	Carrots
	Celery
	Collard greens
	Onion
	Mushrooms
	Parsley
	Cucumber
	Zucchini
	Tomato
	Any veggie of your choice
Starch/Legumes	Quinoa
	Gluten-free oatmeal
	Lentils
	Wild rice
	Black beans
	Chickpeas
	Kidney beans
	Navy beans
	Pinto beans
	Pumpkin
	Squash
	Sweet potato

FOOD GROUP	PREFERRED
Protein	Wild salmon
	Grass-fed beef
	Protein powder with low sugar (less than 5 gm)
	Chicken breast
	Scallops
	Sardines
	Eggs
	Bison
	Lamb
Fats	Avocado
	Walnuts
	Almond
	Macadamia nut oil
	Wild salmon
	Sardine
	Olive oil
	Olives
Fruits	Blackberries
	Blueberries
	Raspberries
	Strawberries
	Peaches
	Grapefruit
	Oranges
	Lemon
	Limes
	Cranberries
	Nectarines
	Guava
	Passion fruit

Restoration Phase:
Seven-Day Sample Menu (for Days 1–30)

To be a champ, you have to believe in yourself when nobody else will.
—Sugar Ray Robinson

Day 1, Monday

Breakfast
Plant-based protein shake

1/2 cup of berries

1/2 avocado

Lunch
Grilled chicken salad with red wine vinaigrette

Handful of almonds

Dinner
Roasted vegetables

4 to 6 ounces salmon

1/3 cup brown rice

Daily Progress Tracker

Daily sugar intake target: 30 to 40 grams

Daily calories: _____

Breakfast: • Sugar: • Calories:	Stress mastery: • Meditation • _____ • _____
Snack (optional): • Sugar: • Calories:	Gratitude log (3 things you are grateful for today): • _____ • _____ • _____
Lunch: • Sugar: • Calories:	Next day action plan: • _____ • _____ • _____ • _____
Snack (optional): • Sugar: • Calories:	Notes: • _____ • _____
Dinner: • Sugar: • Calories:	• _____ • _____ • _____
Snacks (optional): • Sugar: • Calories:	• _____ • _____ • _____
Water	• _____
Other drinks: • Sugar: • Calories:	• _____ • _____ • _____

Life is a great big canvas; throw all the paint you can on it.
—Danny Kaye

Day 2, Tuesday

Breakfast
Gluten-free oatmeal with almond milk
(alternative: coconut milk)
Handful almonds or walnuts

Lunch
Tuna salad
Small apple

Dinner
Garden salad
4 to 6 ounces grilled chicken breast
Small baked sweet potato

Daily Progress Tracker

Daily sugar intake target: 30 to 40 grams

Daily calories: _____

Breakfast: • Sugar: • Calories:	Stress mastery: • Meditation • _____ • _____
Snack (optional): • Sugar: • Calories:	Gratitude log (3 things you are grateful for today): • _____ • _____ • _____
Lunch: • Sugar: • Calories:	Next day action plan: • _____ • _____ • _____ • _____
Snack (optional): • Sugar: • Calories:	Notes: • _____ • _____
Dinner: • Sugar: • Calories:	• _____ • _____ • _____
Snacks (optional): • Sugar: • Calories:	• _____ • _____ • _____
Water	• _____
Other drinks: • Sugar: • Calories:	• _____ • _____ • _____

Winners are ordinary people with extraordinary determination.
—Unknown

Day 3, Wednesday

Breakfast
Kale and spinach egg omelet

Lunch
Roasted Veggie Chickpea Salad

Dinner
Salad bowl
1/2 cup of quinoa
4 ounces of lamb chops

Roasted Veggie Chickpea Salad

Serves 6–8

Ingredients:

3 bunches arugula leaves or mixed greens
2 1/2 cups butternut squash, peeled and diced
5 peeled and precooked beets (or roast beets yourself), chopped
1 (15-ounce) can chickpeas, rinsed and drained
1 pint cherry or plum tomatoes, halved
1/3 cup extra-virgin olive oil, plus 2 tablespoons
1/4 cup freshly squeezed orange juice
kosher salt and freshly ground pepper, to taste

Directions:

1. Preheat oven to 400 degrees.
2. Toss cubed butternut squash with 2 tablespoons olive oil and season generously with salt and pepper.
3. Spread out on a baking sheet in an even layer and bake for 45–50 minutes, or until fork tender.
4. Transfer butternut squash to a large (serving) bowl and add chopped beets, arugula, and halved tomatoes. Add in chickpeas.
5. In a small bowl or glass, whisk together olive oil and orange juice until combined.
6. Drizzle salad dressing over peas and vegetables and gently toss together until everything is coated.
7. Taste and adjust seasoning, if necessary, and serve immediately. Note: if roasting beets at home, place beets in a baking dish with 1/2 cup water. Cover with aluminum foil and bake at 400 degrees for 50–60 minutes, or until fork tender. Let cool before peeling.

Daily Progress Tracker

Daily sugar intake target: 30 to 40 grams

Daily calories: _____

Breakfast: • Sugar: • Calories:	Stress mastery: • Meditation • _____ • _____
Snack (optional): • Sugar: • Calories:	Gratitude log (3 things you are grateful for today): • _____ • _____ • _____
Lunch: • Sugar: • Calories:	Next day action plan: • _____ • _____ • _____ • _____
Snack (optional): • Sugar: • Calories:	Notes: • _____ • _____
Dinner: • Sugar: • Calories:	• _____ • _____ • _____
Snacks (optional): • Sugar: • Calories:	• _____ • _____ • _____
Water	• _____
Other drinks: • Sugar: • Calories:	• _____ • _____ • _____

Above all, be the heroine of your life, not the victim.
—Nora Ephron

Day 4, Thursday

Breakfast
Plant-based protein shake +
almond butter + 1 small banana + ice
Blend into a breakfast smoothie.

Lunch
Cucumber Tomato Salad

Dinner
Roasted vegetables
4–6 ounces of grilled chicken breast
1/3 cup of brown rice

Cucumber Tomato Salad

Ingredients:

18 capri tomatoes or 2 pints large cherry tomatoes, halved
1 cucumber
1/2 small white or red onion, finely chopped, or 4 scallions, thinly
    sliced, or 2 spring onions, very thinly sliced
1/4 cup flat-leaf parsley, chopped
handful basil leaves, torn or cut into chiffonade (shreds)
3 tablespoons extra-virgin olive oil
salt and pepper

Directions:

Combine ingredients in shallow dish and let stand 30 minutes
before serving.

Daily Progress Tracker

Daily sugar intake target: 30 to 40 grams

Daily calories: _____

Breakfast: • Sugar: • Calories:	Stress mastery: • Meditation • _____ • _____
Snack (optional): • Sugar: • Calories:	Gratitude log (3 things you are grateful for today): • _____ • _____ • _____
Lunch: • Sugar: • Calories:	Next day action plan: • _____ • _____ • _____ • _____
Snack (optional): • Sugar: • Calories:	Notes: • _____ • _____
Dinner: • Sugar: • Calories:	• _____ • _____ • _____
Snacks (optional): • Sugar: • Calories:	• _____ • _____ • _____
Water	• _____
Other drinks: • Sugar: • Calories:	• _____ • _____ • _____

Be thankful for what you have; you'll end up having more. If you concentrate on what you don't have, you will never, ever have enough.
—Oprah Winfrey

Day 5, Friday

Breakfast
Gluten-free oatmeal with almond milk
1/2 cup of berries

Lunch
Grilled chicken salad
Small apple (or equivalent fruit)

Dinner
Garden salad
4 to 6 ounces of grilled salmon
Small baked sweet potato

Daily Progress Tracker

Daily sugar intake target: 30 to 40 grams

Daily calories: _____

Breakfast: • Sugar: • Calories:	Stress mastery: • Meditation • _____ • _____
Snack (optional): • Sugar: • Calories:	Gratitude log (3 things you are grateful for today): • _____ • _____ • _____
Lunch: • Sugar: • Calories:	Next day action plan: • _____ • _____ • _____ • _____
Snack (optional): • Sugar: • Calories:	Notes: • _____ • _____
Dinner: • Sugar: • Calories:	• _____ • _____ • _____
Snacks (optional): • Sugar: • Calories:	• _____ • _____ • _____
Water	• _____
Other drinks: • Sugar: • Calories:	• _____ • _____ • _____

Strength and growth come only through continuous effort.
—Napoleon Hill

Day 6, Saturday

Breakfast
Scrambled eggs
1/2 avocado
1/2 cup berries

Lunch
Greek Lentil Salad

Dinner
Roasted Cauliflower Steaks

Greek Lentil Salad

Ingredients:

1/2 cup lentils
1/2 cup quinoa
1 pint grape or cherry tomatoes, halved
2 small/medium zucchini or 1 large, cubed
1/2 cup red onion, finely chopped
1/3 cup kalamata olives, halved and pitted
4 tablespoons chopped fresh oregano
1/2 teaspoon salt
1/4 teaspoon freshly ground black pepper
2 tablespoons fresh lemon juice
6 tablespoon extra-virgin olive oil

Directions:

1. Rinse and drain the lentils.
2. Place in saucepan and cover with 2 inches water.
3. Bring to boil, reduce heat to low, and cover. Simmer 20–25 minutes, until tender. Strain and set aside.
4. While the lentils are cooking, make the quinoa.
5. Place quinoa in a small sauce pot with 1 cup water. Bring to a boil, cover, and simmer until all water is absorbed, about 12 minutes.
6. Remove from heat, keep the lid on, and let sit another 2–3 minutes. Fluff with a fork and set aside.
7. Once the lentils and quinoa have cooled, place in a bowl with the tomatoes, zucchini, red onion, and olives.
8. Whisk together the oregano, salt, ground pepper, lemon juice, and olive oil. Toss with salad.

Roasted Cauliflower Steaks

Serves 6

Ingredients:

1 head cauliflower, medium-sized
3 tablespoons olive oil
1 teaspoon garlic, minced
kosher salt

Directions:

1. Preheat oven to 350 degrees and cover a baking sheet with parchment paper.
2. Stir together the olive oil and garlic. Carefully slice the cauliflower into 1–1 1/2-inch slices. The slices from the center will easily stay in one piece. Keep the outer slices whole as well. Brush both sides with garlic and oil mixture.
3. Season both sides of the slices with salt.
4. Place the cauliflower "steaks" on the parchment-lined pan with the best-looking side up.
5. Bake for 40 minutes or until the center of the cauliflower is tender when pierced with a knife and the exterior is golden brown.

Daily Progress Tracker

Daily sugar intake target: 30 to 40 grams

Daily calories: _____

Breakfast: • Sugar: • Calories:	Stress mastery: • Meditation • _____ • _____
Snack (optional): • Sugar: • Calories:	Gratitude log (3 things you are grateful for today): • _____ • _____ • _____
Lunch: • Sugar: • Calories:	Next day action plan: • _____ • _____ • _____ • _____
Snack (optional): • Sugar: • Calories:	Notes: • _____ • _____
Dinner: • Sugar: • Calories:	• _____ • _____ • _____
Snacks (optional): • Sugar: • Calories:	• _____ • _____ • _____
Water	• _____
Other drinks: • Sugar: • Calories:	• _____ • _____ • _____

*Three grand essentials to happiness in this life are something to do,
something to love, and something to hope for.*
—Joseph Addison

Day 7, Sunday

Breakfast
Protein shake
Piece of fruit
Handful of almonds or walnuts

Lunch
Grilled chicken salad

Dinner
Black Bean and Sweet Potato Hash

Black Bean and Sweet Potato Hash

Serves 2–4
Sugar: 2.78 grams per 1/2 cup

Ingredients:

1 cup chopped onion
1 to 2 cloves garlic, minced
2 cups chopped peeled sweet potatoes
(about 2 small or medium)
2 teaspoons mild or hot chili powder
1/3 cup homemade vegetable broth
1 cup cooked black beans
1/4 cup chopped scallions
splash of hot sauce (optional)
chopped cilantro, for garnish

Directions:

1. Place onions in a nonstick skillet and sauté over medium heat, stirring occasionally, for 2–3 minutes. Add garlic and stir.
2. Add sweet potatoes and chili powder, and stir to coat vegetables with chili powder. Add broth and stir. Cook for about 12 minutes more, stirring occasionally, until potatoes are cooked through. Add more liquid, 1 to 2 tablespoons at a time, as needed, to keep vegetables from sticking to pan.
3. Add the black beans, scallions, and salt. Cook for 1 or 2 minutes more, until beans are heated through.
4. Add hot sauce (if using) and stir. Taste and adjust the seasonings. Top with chopped cilantro and serve.

Daily Progress Tracker

Daily sugar intake target: 30 to 40 grams

Daily calories: _____

Breakfast: • Sugar: • Calories:	Stress mastery: • Meditation • _____ • _____
Snack (optional): • Sugar: • Calories:	Gratitude log (3 things you are grateful for today): • _____ • _____ • _____
Lunch: • Sugar: • Calories:	Next day action plan: • _____ • _____ • _____ • _____
Snack (optional): • Sugar: • Calories:	Notes: • _____ • _____
Dinner: • Sugar: • Calories:	• _____ • _____ • _____
Snacks (optional): • Sugar: • Calories:	• _____ • _____ • _____
Water	• _____
Other drinks: • Sugar: • Calories:	• _____ • _____ • _____

The Maintenance Phase: The Mediterranean Diet

The traditional way of eating throughout the Mediterranean region is more of a lifestyle than a diet. It is a lifestyle that encourages physical activity and enjoying food in the company of friends and family. During the third phase of the program you will eat mostly fresh vegetables and fruits, lean protein, healthy fats, and dairy.

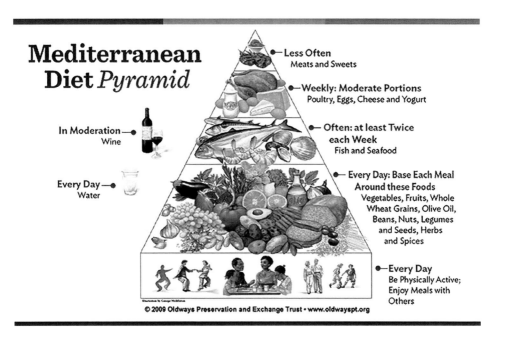

Mediterranean Diet *Pyramid*

Less Often
Meats and Sweets

Weekly: Moderate Portions
Poultry, Eggs, Cheese and Yogurt

Often: at least Twice each Week
Fish and Seafood

In Moderation
Wine

Every Day
Water

Every Day: Base Each Meal Around these Foods
Vegetables, Fruits, Whole Wheat Grains, Olive Oil, Beans, Nuts, Legumes and Seeds, Herbs and Spices

Every Day
Be Physically Active; Enjoy Meals with Others

© 2009 Oldways Preservation and Exchange Trust • www.oldwayspt.org

What to Eat

- **Vegetables:** Enjoy a salad with your main meals. Use olive oil as a dressing. Eat five or more servings of vegetables daily.
- **Fruits:** Eat two or more servings of fruits per day.
- **Whole grains**
- **Legumes**
- **Nuts:** A handful of nuts is healthy. More can work against weight loss because nuts are high in calories.
- **Poultry**
- **Fish**
- **Limited amounts of red meat**
- **Healthy fats such as olive oil and canola oil instead of butter**
- **Herbs and spices instead of salt**
- **Red wine in moderation**

What Not to Eat

- **Refined sugars such as ice cream, candies**
- **Processed food**
- **Processed meat such as hot dogs**
- **Sweetened drinks**
- **Refined carbohydrates**
- **Trans fat**

Mediterranean Diet Sample Menu

Monday, Day 1

Breakfast
Mediterranean Scrambled Eggs with
Spinach, Tomato, and Feta

Lunch
Avocado Tuna Salad

Dinner
Chicken Tandoori with Couscous and Sautéed Green Beans

Mediterranean Scrambled Eggs with Spinach, Tomato, and Feta

Serves 1–2
Preparation time: 2 minutes
Cook time: 4 minutes

Ingredients:

1 tablespoon of olive oil
1/3 cup of tomato, diced and seeded
1/2 cup to 1 cup of spinach
3–4 eggs
2 tablespoons of feta cheese
salt and pepper to taste

Directions:

1. Heat oil in frying pan on medium heat.
2. Sauté the tomatoes and spinach until the spinach wilts.
3. Add eggs and gently mix until scrambled to your liking.
4. Add feta cheese.
5. Season with salt and pepper.

Avocado Tuna Salad (no mayo)

Ingredients:

1 (5 ounce) can of tuna
1 medium avocado
1 carrot, minced
1 stalk of celery, minced
1 tablespoon of lemon juice
1/8 teaspoon of paprika
salt and pepper to taste

Directions

1. Mash tuna and avocado in a bowl.
2. Stir in the remaining ingredients.
3. Serve on a bed of lettuce.

Chicken Tandoori with Couscous and Sautéed Green Beans

Serves 4

Ingredients for chicken tandoori:

3 tablespoons olive oil, divided
1/2 teaspoon cayenne
2 teaspoons ground coriander
1 1/2 teaspoons ground cumin
1 tablespoon garam masala
2 1/2 teaspoons paprika
1 teaspoon ground turmeric
1 15-ounce can full-fat coconut milk
2 tablespoons lemon juice
5 cloves garlic, minced
1 tablespoon fresh ginger, minced
1 teaspoon of salt
black pepper, to taste
6–8 chicken drumsticks or a combination of drumsticks and thighs
    bones (or chicken breast)
1–2 large onions, sliced into rounds
lemon wedges and cilantro, for serving

Directions:

1. Heat oil in a small skillet over medium heat. Add all the spices (through turmeric) and cook, stirring, until fragrant, about 2–3 minutes. Let cool completely.
2. In a medium bowl, whisk together coconut milk with spices. Stir in garlic, ginger, lemon, salt, and pepper.
3. Coat chicken in marinade. Cover and chill at least 3 hours or overnight.

4. When ready to cook, preheat oven to 350 degrees and line a baking sheet with foil. Transfer chicken to baking sheet, reserving excess marinade. Bake for 20 minutes, then generously brush on extra marinade. Bake another 10 minutes, remove, and generously brush on more marinade. Bake a final 10–15 minutes or until chicken is cooked all the way through.
5. Meanwhile, in a large skillet, heat the final tablespoon of olive oil over medium-high heat. Add onion rounds. Cover and cook 3 minutes. Flip, cover, and cook 3 minutes more.
6. Serve chicken with cooked onions, lemon wedges, and cilantro.

Ingredients for couscous:

1/3 cup water
1/2 cup instant couscous
2 tablespoons chopped fresh parsley
1/2 teaspoon paprika
1/8 teaspoon turmeric
1 tablespoon lemon juice
1/8 teaspoon kosher salt
pinch of black pepper
1 tablespoon olive oil

Directions for couscous:

1. In a small skillet, heat a drizzle of olive oil over medium heat.
2. In a small saucepan, bring 1/3 cup of water to a boil.
3. Add 1/2 cup of instant couscous. Turn off the heat and let set, covered, for 2–3 minutes.
4. Chop parsley leaves into 2 tablespoons.
5. Remove the lid and stir in 1/2 teaspoon paprika, 1/8 teaspoon turmeric, 1 tablespoon lemon juice, the parsley, 1/8 teaspoon kosher salt, pinch of black pepper, and 1 tablespoon olive oil. Return the lid and let set for another 2–3 minutes.

Ingredients for sautéed green beans:

2 cups of green beans, trimmed
1 tablespoon of ghee or olive oil
salt and ground black pepper

Directions:

1. In a skillet, sauté the green beans in butter until tender-crisp.
Season with salt and black pepper, to taste.

Tuesday, Day 2

Breakfast
Three Ingredient Pancakes

Lunch
Spinach Salad with Feta, Apples, and Walnuts

Dinner
Mediterranean Turkey Burger with
Caramelized Onions and Sweet Potato Fries

Three Ingredient Pancakes

Serves 1

Ingredients:

1 medium ripe banana
2 tablespoons whole-wheat flour
1 large egg, lightly beaten

Directions:

1. Mash banana with a fork until smooth. Add flour and egg; stir
   well with a whisk.
2. Heat a large nonstick skillet or griddle over medium-high heat.
   Spoon batter onto skillet, using one-third of batter for each
   pancake.
3. Cook 2 minutes or until tops are covered with bubbles and edges
   look cooked. Carefully turn pancakes over; cook 1 to 2 minutes
   or until bottoms are lightly browned.

Spinach Salad with Feta, Apples and Walnuts

Serves 4

Ingredients:

8 cups baby spinach, washed
1 apple, cored and thinly sliced
1/2 cup chopped walnuts
1/4 cup apple balsamic vinegar
3 tablespoons extra virgin olive oil
kosher salt and black pepper, to taste
1/2 cup feta cheese

Directions:

1. Add cleaned spinach to a bowl; then top with sliced apples and pecans.
2. Whisk together the vinegar, oil, salt, and pepper; then pour over the salad (or place in a separate dispenser for later).
3. Add feta.

Mediterranean Turkey Burger with Caramelized Onions and Sweet Potato Fries

Serves 4

Ingredients:

1 pound ground turkey

1/4 cup feta cheese (fat-free works too), crumbled

1/4 cup pesto, prepared

2 onions—only white and light parts—thinly sliced and
   sautéed in 1 tablespoon ghee or olive oil in a frying pan
   to a caramelized color.

Directions:

1. Mix together all ingredients until uniform.
2. Form 3 patties, each 3/4 inch thick.
3. Grill on one side for 3–5 minutes, then flip and cook until meat
   is fully cooked.
4. Serve with caramelized onions or any Mediterranean toppings.

Wednesday, Day 3

Breakfast
Cinnamon Apple Quinoa

Lunch
Grilled Hummus Veggie Wraps

Dinner
Lemon Rosemary Salmon with Three Bean Salad

Cinnamon Apple Quinoa

Serves 4

Ingredients:

1 cup dry quinoa, rinsed well
1 1/2 cups water
1 teaspoon cinnamon + more for sprinkling
2 teaspoons vanilla extract
1/2 cup unsweetened applesauce
1/4 cup golden raisins
1 cup warmed almond milk
1 gala apple, peeled and diced
1/4 cup walnuts, chopped

Directions:

1. Combine quinoa, water, cinnamon, and vanilla in a small saucepan and bring to boil.
2. Reduce to a simmer, cover, and let cook for 15 minutes until quinoa can be fluffed with a fork.
3. Divide cooked quinoa between four bowls, then stir in applesauce and raisins, and pour in warmed milk.
4. Top with fresh cut apples and walnuts and a dash of cinnamon.

Grilled Hummus Veggie Wraps

Serves 2

Ingredients:

1 zucchini, ends removed, sliced
salt and pepper to taste
1 tablespoon olive oil
1 tomato, sliced, or a handful of cherry tomatoes
1/8 cup sliced red onion
1 cup kale, tough stems removed
2 slices white cheddar or chipotle gouda cheese
2 large gluten-free tortillas
4 tablespoons hummus

Directions:

1. Heat a skillet or grill to medium heat.
2. Remove the ends from the zucchini and slice lengthwise into strips. Toss sliced zucchini in olive oil and sprinkle with salt and pepper.
3. Place sliced zucchini directly on grill and let cook for 3 minutes; turn and cook for 2 more minutes.
4. Set zucchini aside.
5. Place the tortillas on the grill for approximately one minute, or just until grill marks are visible and tortillas are pliable.
6. Remove the tortillas from the grill and assemble wraps, 2 tablespoons of hummus, one slice of cheese, zucchini slices, 1/2 cup of kale, onion, and tomato slices.
7. Wrap tightly.

Lemon Rosemary Salmon with Three Bean Salad

Serves 3

Ingredients for salmon:

1 pound salmon fillet
1 tablespoon olive oil
1/3 cup dry white wine (optional)
1/8 cup lemon juice
1 tablespoon honey
1/2 tablespoon finely chopped fresh rosemary leaves
1 teaspoon almond flour (used as a thickener)
salt, pepper
lemon slices and rosemary to garnish

Directions:

1. Cut the salmon fillet into the serving-sized pieces.
2. Sprinkle the salmon with salt and pepper, and brush the top with olive oil.
3. Heat up a large, nonstick skillet on medium heat. Add the salmon to the pan, skin side up, cover with lid, and cook for about 3–4 minutes.
4. After 4 minutes, flip the salmon and cook for another 3 minutes. Remove salmon from the pan and set aside.
5. To the same pan add wine, lemon juice, honey, and rosemary. Stir and cook for about 2 minutes.
6. Add the almond flour into the sauce. Cook for another minute and add the salmon to the pan, skin side up. Turn off the heat, cover the dish with a lid, and let it rest for a few minutes.
7. Flip the salmon before serving and garnish with lemon slices and fresh rosemary.

Ingredients for three bean salad:

1 can (8 ounces) cut green beans, drained
1 can (8 ounces) cut wax beans, drained
3/4 cup canned kidney beans, rinsed and drained
1/4 cup chopped onion
2 tablespoons honey
2 tablespoons white vinegar
1 tablespoon canola oil
1/8 teaspoon pepper

Directions:

In a small bowl, combine the first four ingredients. In another bowl, whisk the honey, vinegar, oil and pepper; stir into the bean mixture. Cover and refrigerate until serving.

Thursday, Day 4

Breakfast
Kale and Sweet Potato Breakfast Cups

Lunch
Mediterranean Cobb Salad

Dinner
Grass-Fed Steak with Mushroom Sauce,
and Oven Roasted Asparagus and Brussels Sprouts

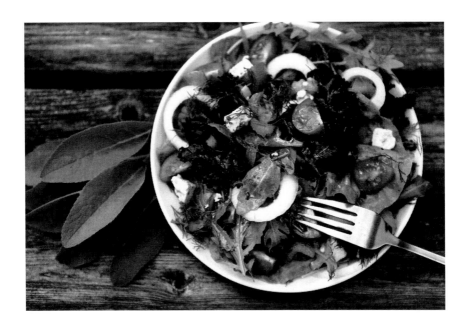

Kale and Sweet Potato Breakfast Cups

Serves 4

Ingredients:

1-second spray of olive oil
11 large eggs
1/2 teaspoon salt
1 tablespoon olive oil, extra virgin
3/4 raw sweet potato
1/3 cup red onion
1 1/2 ounce baby kale
1/2 cup crumbled goat cheese
2 tablespoons basil, fresh

Directions:

1. Preheat oven to 375 degrees.
2. Spritz the 12 cups of a nonstick muffin tray with cooking spray.
3. In a large bowl, whisk together the eggs and salt. Set aside.
4. Heat the oil in a medium or large stick-resistant skillet over medium-high heat. Add sweet potato and onion and sauté until they begin to brown, about 5 minutes.
5. Add kale, remove from heat, and stir until kale is fully wilted.
6. Add sweet potato-kale mixture to egg mixture and quickly stir. Add the goat cheese and basil and stir until evenly combined.
7. Ladle the egg mixture into the muffin cups, filling each about 7/8 full.
8. Bake until the egg frittata cups are just set, about 18 minutes. Remove from the muffin tray and serve while warm.

Mediterranean Cobb Salad

Serves 2

Ingredients for the salad:

4 cups romaine lettuce
1 to 2 hard boiled eggs, thinly sliced
2 cups artichoke hearts
1 cup marinated roasted red peppers, drained
3/4 cup cucumbers, diced into small pieces
3/4 cup feta cheese, crumbled or diced small
1/2 cup olives (black olives or kalamata)
2 tablespoons fresh basil, for garnishing

Ingredients for the vinaigrette:

3 to 4 tablespoons olive oil
1 to 2 tablespoons balsamic or red wine vinegar
1 tablespoon honey, or to taste
1/2 teaspoon dried oregano
1/2 teaspoon dried basil
1/2 teaspoon dried dill
1/2 teaspoon kosher salt, or to taste
1/2 teaspoon freshly ground black pepper, or to taste

Directions:

1. Salad: In a large serving platter, evenly scatter the romaine, evenly lay down the remaining ingredients in long rows, and evenly sprinkle with fresh basil; set aside.
2. Vinaigrette: Whisk ingredients together and drizzle over salad and serve immediately.

Grass-Fed Steak with Mushroom Sauce, and Oven Roasted Asparagus and Brussels Sprouts

Serves 6

Ingredients for steaks:

2 tablespoons ghee
four 4-ounce packages gourmet blend mushrooms, sliced
4 cloves garlic, minced
1 shallot, minced
1 cup beef broth
1/2 cup of coconut cream
1/2 teaspoon dried thyme
salt and fresh ground black pepper
six 1-inch-thick rib eye steaks
2 tablespoons olive oil
fresh thyme leaves, for garnish, optional

Directions:

1. In a large skillet, melt the ghee over medium heat. Add the mushrooms, garlic, and shallots. Cook, stirring frequently, until the mushrooms are tender, about 10 minutes.
2. Add the broth and bring to a boil. Reduce the heat and simmer until the liquid is reduced to about 1/2 cup, about 12 minutes.
3. Stir in the cream and simmer until the sauce is thickened, 6 to 8 minutes. Stir in the thyme, 1/2 teaspoon salt, and 1/2 teaspoon pepper. Set aside and keep warm.
4. Sprinkle the steaks evenly with salt and pepper.
5. In a large skillet, heat the oil over medium-high heat. Add the steaks, in batches if necessary, and cook for 4 to 5 minutes per side or until desired degree of being done.

6. Remove from the skillet and let stand for 10 minutes.
7. Serve the steaks with the mushroom sauce. Garnish with thyme leaves if desired.

Ingredients for asparagus and Brussels sprouts:

1 bunch of asparagus, cleaned
1 pound small brussels sprouts, cut in half and cleaned
1 teaspoon salt
1 teaspoon pepper
4 tablespoon olive oil

Directions:

1. Preheat oven to 450 degrees.
2. Put cleaned asparagus on cookie sheet and spread out in one even layer.
3. Pour about 2 tablespoons olive oil over asparagus and sprinkle with half the salt and pepper.
4. Put cleaned brussels sprouts in a bowl and drizzle remaining olive oil over them. Stir brussels sprouts around in the bowl until they are all evenly coated. Spread them out on a cookie sheet with asparagus.
5. Sprinkle remaining salt and pepper over the brussels sprouts.
6. Move the asparagus and brussels sprouts around the tray a little to ensure even coating of oil and seasonings.
7. Cook for 30–45 minutes at 450 degrees until the asparagus and brussels sprouts are done to your liking.

Friday, Day 5

Breakfast
Breakfast Scramble Stuffed Avocado

Lunch
Grilled Zucchini Pizza

Dinner
Spicy Shrimp Bowl with Parmesan Quinoa and Garlic Kale

Breakfast Scramble
Stuffed Avocado

Serves 1

Ingredients:

1 ripe avocado
sea salt to taste
1 tablespoon ghee
2 extra-large whole eggs
1 ounce shredded mozzarella cheese
1 ounce turkey bacon, finely diced
quartered heirloom tomatoes for serving
fresh herbs (parsley, chives, or basil) for topping
black pepper, to serve

Directions:

1. Prepare avocado first by halving, pitting, and then gently peeling to remove skin. Scoop out some of the avocado flesh, leaving a 1/4-inch edge around it to create a "boat." Season with salt and set aside.
2. Fry the bacon pieces in a nonstick pan until golden and crisp; transfer to a warm plate.
3. Lightly whisk the eggs. Melt the butter over low-medium heat in the same nonstick pan. As it begins to bubble, add the eggs and stir them around until just starting to cook through. Cook the eggs to your preferred consistency, remove from heat, and add the cheese, folding it through the eggs until the cheese has melted. Spoon into the prepared avocado boats.
4. Season with the crispy bacon, herbs, and pepper. Serve with tomatoes.

Grilled Zucchini Pizza

Serves 4

Ingredients:

1 large zucchini
1/4 cup ghee (melted) or olive oil
3 cloves crushed garlic
1/2 cup mozzarella cheese
14 ounces white or red sauce
topping of your choice

Directions:

1. Slice the zucchini into thick rounds. Combine the melted butter and crushed garlic in a small bowl. Set aside.
2. When the coals on your barbecue are almost burned down, lay your zucchini slices on the grill. Let cook for 3 minutes, then turn over and lightly brush the butter/garlic mixture on each slice. Cook for 3 more minutes and turn over again and lightly brush the other side with the garlic and butter. (Can also use same method in lightly oiled frying pan.)
3. Cover the slices with pizza sauce and cheese and let cook and add toppings. DONE when cheese begins to melt.

Spicy Shrimp Bowl with Parmesan Quinoa and Garlic Kale

Ingredients:

1 cup cooked quinoa (about 1/2 cup dry quinoa to 1 cup of stock)
6 large white shrimp, peeled and deveined
1/4 teaspoon chili powder
1/4 teaspoon garlic powder
1/4 teaspoon salt
1/8 teaspoon cayenne pepper
1 cup kale, fibrous stems removed and leaves chopped into bite size pieces
1 clove garlic, minced
1/4 cup grated Parmesan cheese
2 teaspoons olive oil

Directions:

1. Cook quinoa according to package instructions.
2. Mix spices together in a small bowl and season both sides of the shrimp with the mixture.
3. Heat a skillet over medium high heat with 1 teaspoon olive oil.
4. Sear shrimp on both sides until browned and cooked through.
5. Remove shrimp and turn your skillet down to medium/ medium low.
6. Add your remaining 1 teaspoon of olive oil and your minced garlic.
7. Sauté garlic on low heat for a few minutes. (Don't burn.)
8. Add in kale on low heat. Stir and let the kale cook down for a few minutes.
9. Add salt and pepper to taste.
10. To your cooked, still-warm quinoa, stir in your Parmesan cheese. Season to taste with salt and pepper.
11. Add quinoa, shrimp, and garlic kale in a bowl.

Saturday, Day 6

Breakfast
Middle Eastern Labneh Hummus Salad (Egg Platter)

Lunch
Roasted Balsamic Beet, Goat Cheese, Pistachio Salad

Dinner
Rosemary Garlic Lamb Chops with
Honey Cider Glaze and Roasted Cauliflower

Middle Eastern Labneh Hummus Salad (Egg Platter)

Serves 1

Ingredients:

1 scoop hummus
sunny-side-up eggs, poached or hardboiled
dates
pickled cucumbers or olives
tomatoes
cucumbers
any kind of vegetables of your choice

Directions:

Assemble on a platter your way.

Roasted Balsamic Beet, Goat Cheese, Pistachio Salad

Serves 2

Ingredients for salad:

5–6 medium to large-sized beets (suggestion: golden and chioggia beets)
2 ounces goat cheese, crumbled
1/4 cup shelled unsalted or salted pistachios
olive oil, kosher salt, and freshly ground black pepper for roasting and finishing the salad

Ingredients for balsamic vinaigrette:

2 tablespoons white or golden balsamic vinegar
2 teaspoon olive oil
1 teaspoon honey
kosher salt and black pepper to taste

Directions:

1. Preheat oven to 400 degrees.
2. Line a rimmed baking sheet with foil.
3. Peel the beets with a vegetable peeler and cut them into wedges.
4. Place the beets on the prepared baking sheet, drizzle them with olive oil, salt, and pepper and toss to coat them.
5. Keep mixed-variety beets separate or they will bleed color.
6. Spread the beets into a single layer then roast them for approximately 25–30 minutes or until tender, shaking the tray and tossing them around a couple of times to ensure even cooking.
7. Remove from the oven and let cool while you make the vinaigrette.
8. Whisk together all of the ingredients for the vinaigrette in a medium-sized bowl.
9. Place the beets in the vinaigrette and toss until coated.

10. Divide the vinaigrette into separate bowls, as the beet juices will dye the vinaigrette.
11. Arrange the beets onto a serving platter or in a bowl and top with crumbled goat cheese, pistachios, kosher salt, and freshly ground black pepper.

Rosemary Garlic Lamb Chops with Honey Cider Glaze and Roasted Cauliflower

Serves 2

Ingredients:

8 lamb chops
salt and freshly ground black pepper
1/4 cup olive oil, plus 1 tablespoon
1 tablespoon minced garlic
2 teaspoons chopped fresh rosemary
1 tablespoon minced shallots
1/2 cup apple cider
1 tablespoon cider vinegar
1 tablespoon honey

Directions:

1. Place the lamb chops in a shallow dish, then season the lamb chops on all sides with salt and pepper. Combine the marinade of 1/4 cup olive oil, garlic, and rosemary in a small bowl or plastic ziploc baggie, then pour over the lamb chops. Marinate the lamb chops in the refrigerator for 1 hour.
2. Heat the remaining tablespoon of olive oil in a large sauté pan over medium-high heat until shimmering. Working in batches, cook the lamb chops in the pan until brown and crusty, 2–3 minutes per side for medium rare. Transfer the lamb chops to a large platter and let rest at room temperature.
3. While lamb rests, add the shallots to the pan and cook, stirring constantly, until the shallots start to soften, 2–3 minutes. Pour the apple cider into the pan, stirring to scrape up any browned

bits from the bottom of the pan. Stir in the vinegar and the honey, bring to a boil, then reduce heat and simmer for 5 minutes until the sauce is slightly thickened. Spoon the glaze over the lamb chops and serve with roasted cauliflower.

Sunday, Day 7

Breakfast
Oatmeal Breakfast Bites

Lunch
Greek Chickpea Salad

Dinner
Grilled salmon, with vegetables and sweet potato

Oatmeal Breakfast Bites

Serves 12

Ingredients:

3 large ripe bananas
1/2 cup of almond butter
1 tablespoon ghee, softened
2 tablespoons agave or honey
1 teaspoon vanilla extract
1 egg, beaten
2 1/2 cups steel cut oats
1 teaspoon baking powder
1/4 teaspoon ground cinnamon
1/4 teaspoon salt
1/2 cup dark chocolate chips
1/4 cup chopped seasonal fruit

Directions:

1. Preheat oven to 350 degrees.
2. In a large bowl, mash the ripe bananas with a fork. Stir in the almond butter, ghee, honey, and vanilla extract and mix until smooth.
3. In a separate medium bowl, stir together the oats, baking powder, cinnamon, and salt.
4. Add the dry ingredients to the wet ingredients and stir until combined.
5. Add the beaten egg and stir until combined.
6. Add in chocolate chips and/or chopped seasonal fruit.
7. Form large, flat cookies by hand and place on a cookie sheet lined with parchment paper.
8. Bake for 15 minutes or until cookies are done.
9. Let cool on baking sheet.

Greek Chickpea Salad

Serves 8

Ingredients for the dressing:

1/2 cup olive oil
1/4 cup lemon juice
1/3 cup chopped fresh parsley
1 teaspoon dried oregano
1/2 teaspoon salt
1/4 teaspoon pepper

Ingredients for the salad:

3 cups chickpeas, drained and rinsed
2 cups halved cherry tomatoes
1 English cucumber, seeded and chopped
1 red bell pepper, chopped
1 small red onion, finely chopped
1/2 cup sliced black olives
1 cup crumbled feta

Directions:

1. In a medium bowl, whisk together dressing ingredients.
2. Combine all salad ingredients in a large bowl.
3. Add the dressing to the salad bowl, and stir to combine.
4. Refrigerate for 15–30 minutes before serving.

Additional Menu Options

Breakfast Options
Protein shake

Yogurt

Oatmeal

Fruit

Cottage cheese

Boiled egg

Omelet

Lunch Options
Soups

Salads

Grilled chicken salad or sandwich

Lettuce wraps with veggies, grilled chicken, turkey, or tuna

Fajitas with chicken

Dinner Options
Soups

Salads

Fish (not fried)

Grilled chicken

Baked potato or yam

Brown rice

Beans and legumes

Gluten-free pasta

Lean pork or steak

Snack Options
Fruits

Yogurt

Veggies

Cottage cheese

Protein shakes

Protein bars

Hummus

Nuts, in limited amounts

Cheese sticks

Roasted chickpeas

Boiled eggs

Celery and peanut butter

Drink Options
Water

Flavored water

Sparkling water

Diet ice tea

Diet sodas

Coffee

Tea

Limit alcohol to no more than one drink a day.

Section 5

Dealing with Special Dieting Challenges

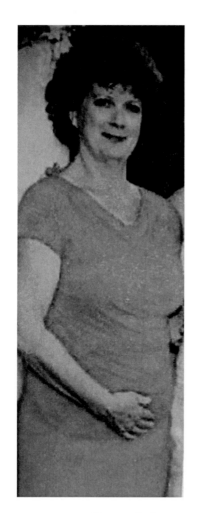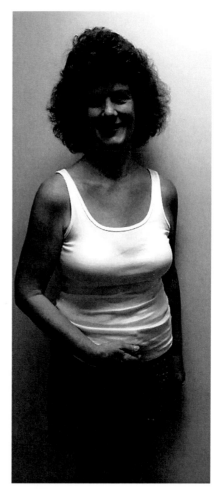

Lost 34 pounds over 4 years.

Our greatest weakness lies in giving up. The most certain way to succeed is always to try just one more time.

—Thomas A. Edison

Preparing for Special Occasions

Sticking to a healthy lifestyle can be challenging, especially during special occasions such as when traveling, holidays, business meetings, and parties. These should be no excuse to give up on yourself. If you have a severe allergy to a food, you will still avoid it during such occasions. This again goes back to the brain associating the culprit food with danger, which will naturally keep you from harm. Try the following to help you stay on course:

1. Plan what you are going to eat ahead of time.
2. Pack what you need, just as you would if you are on a prescription medicine. Think of food as life-saving medicine.
3. At a party, skip the appetizers or have a salad instead.
4. Minimize alcohol intake at parties. Focus on enjoying the company.
5. Eat a healthy snack before you go to a party so you are not that hungry when you get there.
6. At a restaurant, ask for what you want and don't worry about what others are ordering. Remember your body does not care what your friends think or say about your choices. It only cares what you feed it. Focus on what you need to nourish your body, not what they think or want.

The Dreaded Diet Plateau

At some point, you are going to hit a plateau. Everybody does. When you do, don't be frustrated or give up. Use the following tips to get back on track:

- Use a food diary to track your calorie consumption.
- Drink at least eight glasses of water a day.
- Eat breakfast regularly.
- Eat more protein and high-fiber foods.
- Exercise most days of the week.
- Learn to control stress. (Prolonged stress will lead to production of stress hormones such as cortisol, which will make it harder to lose weight.)

Notes:

_____

_____

_____

_____

_____

_____

_____

_____

_____

_____

_____

_____

_____

_____

Section 6

Other Obstacles to Weight Loss

Some medical conditions are known to cause weight gain or make it harder to lose weight. When you are doing everything "right" but the weight just won't come off, you may have a medical problem. When you seem stuck, look for one or more of the following reasons, which I represent here with an acronym:

"CHIEFMUDS"

Carbohydrate sensitivity
Hormonal imbalance
Inactivity
Emotional eating
Food allergy
Metabolic syndrome
Unclear reason
Drug side effects
Sleep disorder

Use the following questionnaire to see if you may have any of these.

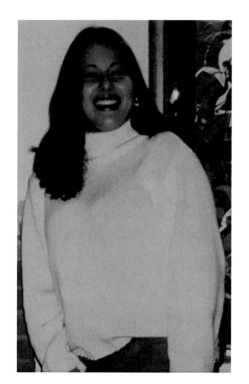 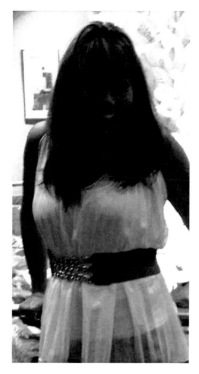

Lost 30 pounds and has kept it off over 4 years.

The CHIEFMUDS
Questionnaire™

Carbohydrate Sensitivity:

Do you feel sluggish after a starchy meal?	(a) Yes (b) No
Do you crave carbohydrates?	(a) Yes (b) No
Do you feel like you are "addicted" to carbs?	(a) Yes (b) No

Hormonal Imbalance:

Hypothyroidism, PCOS, Cushings,
adrenal hypersecretion, low testosterone

Hypothyroidism:

Do you have low energy level?	(a) Yes (b) No
Do you feel excessively cold?	(a) Yes (b) No
Do you have dry skin?	(a) Yes (b) No
Do you have brittle nails?	(a) Yes (b) No
Do feel a bit depressed?	(a) Yes (b) No
Do you have dry hair or hair loss?	(a) Yes (b) No
Do you have high cholesterol?	(a) Yes (b) No
Do you have a family history of hypothyroidism	(a) Yes (b) No

Polycystic Ovary Syndrome (PCOS):

Do you have unwanted facial hair?	(a) Yes (b) No
Do you have infrequent menses?	(a) Yes (b) No
Do you bulk easily with resistance training?	(a) Yes (b) No
Do have thinning of the hair on top of your head?	(a) Yes (b) No
Do you have skin tags or had them removed?	(a) Yes (b) No
Is the skin on the back of your neck darker?	(a) Yes (b) No
Is the skin in your armpits darker?	(a) Yes (b) No

Adrenal Hypersecretion:

Are you under a lot of stress?	(a) Yes (b) No
Are you retaining fluids?	(a) Yes (b) No
Do you have borderline high glucose?	(a) Yes (b) No
Do you have borderline high blood pressure?	(a) Yes (b) No
Do you have a hump on the lower neck area?	(a) Yes (b) No

Inactivity:

How many hours a day do you spend watching TV?
(a) less than 1   (b) 1–2   (c) more than 2

How many hours a week do you do yard or house work or duties on the job that cause you to work up a sweat?
(a) 4 or more   (b) 1–3   (c) Less than one

How many times a week do you get out for a brisk walk of 10 minutes or more?
(a) 4 or more   (b) 1–3   (c) Less than 1

How many times a week do you participate in sports or an exercise program?
(a) 4 or more   (b) 1–3   (c) Less than 1

Emotional Eating:

How often do you eat when you are not hungry but because of stress or for emotional reasons?
(a) Rarely   (b) Sometimes   (c) Often   (d) All the time

Food Allergies:

Do you have a history of allergies most of your life?	(a) Yes (b) No
Did you have colic as an infant?	(a) Yes (b) No
Do you have frequent sinus or ear infections?	(a) Yes (b) No
Do you have eczema?	(a) Yes (b) No
Do you have frequent hives?	(a) Yes (b) No

Do you have asthma?   (a) Yes (b) No

Do you have irritable bowel syndrome?   (a) Yes (b) No

Do you have frequent headaches?   (a) Yes (b) No

Metabolic Syndrome:

Do you have erratic energy?   (a) Yes (b) No

Do you have mood swings that can be
affected by eating?   (a) Yes (b) No

Do you have unwanted facial hair?   (a) Yes (b) No

Do you have a history of difficulty
getting pregnant?   (a) Yes (b) No

Do you have history of ovarian cysts?   (a) Yes (b) No

Do you have borderline high glucose?   (a) Yes (b) No

Do you have history of high blood pressure?   (a) Yes (b) No

Do you have a history of high triglycerides?   (a) Yes (b) No

Do you have a history of diabetes during
pregnancy?   (a) Yes (b) No

Sleep Disorder:

Do you have a snoring problem?   (a) Yes (b) No

Do you nap during the day?   (a) Yes (b) No

Do you have trouble staying awake during the day?   (a) Yes (b) No

Has anyone noticed irregular breathing while
you are asleep?   (a) Yes (b) No

How many hours of sleep do you get a night? _____

Drug Side Effects:

Are you taking any of the following medications?

    Lyrica   (a) Yes (b) No

    Depakote   (a) Yes (b) No

    Remeron   (a) Yes (b) No

SSRIs such as Paxil, Lexapro, Celexa	(a) Yes	(b) No
Antidepressants such as amitriptyline and trazodone	(a) Yes	(b) No
Prednisone	(a) Yes	(b) No
Lithium	(a) Yes	(b) No
Birth control pills with ethinylestradiol	(a) Yes	(b) No
Insulin	(a) Yes	(b) No
Glucotrol or glipizide	(a) Yes	(b) No
Actos	(a) Yes	(b) No
Clozapine	(a) Yes	(b) No
Olanzapine	(a) Yes	(b) No
Haldol	(a) Yes	(b) No
Arimidex	(a) Yes	(b) No
Others	(a) Yes	(b) No

The CHIEFMUDS Action Plan

Suggestions for Carbohydrate Sensitivity:
Protein-based meals and snacks
Frequent small meals
Low glycemic index carbohydrates
Do not skip breakfast
Increase fiber
Cinnamon, lemon juice and vinegar, chromium

Suggestions for Hypothyroidism:
Discuss with your healthcare provider about getting labs:
    TSH, Free T3 and T4
Treat as appropriate

Suggestions for Emotional Eating:
Exercise
Rejuvenation list
Humor
Small dishes
Change routine
Use techniques discussed earlier

Suggestions for Food Allergies:
Allergy panel
Elimination diet

Suggestions for Metabolic Syndrome:
Modified Mediterranean diet
Small frequent meals (six meals per day)
Exercise
Chromium
Cinnamon

Green tea
Vitamins C, E
Alpha lipoic acid
Fish oil with EPA and DHA
Multivitamin

Suggestions for Drug Side Effects:
Weight-neutral alternative whenever possible

Suggestions for Sleep Disorder:
Sleep hygiene
Treat sleep apnea
Treat insomnia

---

* **Sleep hygiene** refers to practices and routines that help you to get a restful night's sleep. If you struggle to get a good night's sleep, try some of the following;
    - Have a consistent bedtime
    - Avoid stimulants such as caffeine within 3 hours of bedtime
    - Your bedroom should be at a comfortable temperature: around 65 to 68 degrees Fahrenheit
    - Have a relaxing bedtime routine such as taking a bath or reading a book
    - Avoid daytime napping
    - No TV or electronic gadgets in the bedroom
    - Avoid strenuous exercise too close to bedtime
    - If you are in bed but not asleep after 30 minutes, get out of the bedroom and do something relaxing until you are ready to fall asleep

Section 7

Other Resources

More about the Main Food Groups

There are three main classes of foods. These are carbohydrates, protein, and fats.

Carbohydrates **are starchy foods.** Examples are bread, pasta, rice, vegetables, and fruits. They have high starch content and are broken down after digestion into sugar. Carbohydrates provide the fuel that the brain, muscles, and tissues need to function. There are about four calories per gram of carbohydrate.

Not all carbohydrates are created equal. Choosing good carbohydrates is more likely to support your weight-loss efforts. What are good carbohydrates? When we eat carbohydrates, they are broken down into sugar. The impact of any food on blood sugar is measured by what is called the glycemic index.

The Glycemic Index

The Glycemic Index (GI) is a measure of the impact of a given food on blood glucose level. The higher the glycemic index, the faster a given amount of that food raises the level of blood glucose. Conversely, food with a lower glycemic index will produce slower and lower spikes in blood glucose levels. Glucose is used as the standard of comparison and it has a score of 100. A food is classified as low GI if it has a score of 55 or less. Medium GI is a score of 56 to 69 and a high GI is a score of 70 or higher.

A food that has a high glycemic index will cause a rapid spike in blood sugar. The body responds by making very high levels of the hormone insulin to help lower the blood sugar. Over time the levels of insulin can become persistently elevated, a condition called hyperinsulinemia. Excess insulin leads to an increase in fat accumulation

127

and has been associated with heart disease, elevated triglycerides, and metabolic syndrome.

If you want to lose weight it is important to choose foods that have low glycemic indexes. This is particularly important if you have diabetes. The following is a partial list of commonly available foods and their glycemic indexes. The goal is to select foods from the green zone.

Glycemic Index Guide

Type of food	Low		Medium		High	
	Food	GI Score	Food	GI Score	Food	GI Score
Vegetables	Carrots	49	Beets	64	Parsnips	97
	Green peas	48	Fresh corn	60	Pumpkin	75
	Broccoli	15				
	Eggplant	15				
	Spinach	15				
	Tomatoes	15				
	Zucchini	15				
	Cabbage	10				
	Lettuce	10				
	Mushrooms	10				
	Onions	10				
	Red peppers	10				
Fruits	Kiwi	52	Pineapple	66	Dates	103
	Grapes	46	Raisins	64	Watermelon	80
	Oranges	44	Figs	61		
	Peaches	42	Mango	60		
	Strawberries	40	Banana	58		

Type of food	Low		Medium		High	
	Food	GI Score	Food	GI Score	Food	GI Score
	Apples	38				
	Plums	38				
	Pears	37				
	Grapefruit	25				
	Cherries	22				
Breakfast foods	Oat and raisin bread	54	Wheat bread	68	Cornflakes	83
	Special K	54	Shredded wheat	67	Corn Chex	83
	All-Bran	51	Croissant	67	Total cereal	76
	Oatmeal	48	Rye bread	64	Cheerios	74
					Raisin bran	73
					Plain bagel	72
					White bread	70
Other carbs	Wheat pasta	54	Taco shells	68	Rice pasta	92
	Yams	54	Cornmeal	68	Instant white rice	87
	Brown rice	50	Baked potato	60	Instant mashed potatoes	80
	Navy beans	38	Wild rice	57	French fries	75
	Black beans	30			Tapioca	70
	Red lentils	27				
	Soy	16				

The second class of food is *protein*. Examples include meat, poultry, eggs, and legumes. Each gram of protein provides four calories. Proteins are needed as building blocks for cells and are important for proper immune function.

If you are trying to lose weight or to keep weight off, adding high-quality protein while lowering refined carbohydrates is a way to ensure that you lose mostly fat and not muscle. Increasing the consumption of high quality protein has been shown to have a lot of benefits, including the following:

Weight loss/fat loss
Energy increase
Immune function boost
Gaining of lean muscle mass
Heart disease prevention
Thermogenesis, or calorie-burning increase
Lower insulin levels in the blood
Osteoporosis prevention
Stabilizing of blood sugar
Satiation—feeling full longer because the food stays longer in the
    stomach

All proteins are not created equal. High-quality protein is complete protein, that is, it contains the nine essential amino acids that are needed by humans. Some good sources of high-quality protein include poultry, fish, beef, eggs, yogurt, and milk. Plant proteins do not contain all the essential amino acids our bodies need. To get all nine essential amino acids from plant sources alone requires eating a combination of foods. Plant sources of protein include nuts, whole grains, and vegetables.

The third class of food is *fats*. They provide the body with essential fatty acids and allow us to properly use fat soluble vitamins.

Each gram of fat provides about nine calories. Fats are calorie dense. A diet that is relatively high in fat will therefore have high calories and may lead to excess weight.

There are four main types of fat, as follows:

1. Saturated fat. Sources include animal fat such as red meat, whole milk dairy products, ice cream, butter, and sour cream. Plant sources include coconut oil, cocoa butter, and palm oil.
2. Monounsaturated fat. This is considered good fat because it has been shown to have a salutary effect on the heart. Good sources include olive oil, canola oil, vegetable oil, nuts, and avocados. These should be consumed in moderation because they are calorie dense.
3. Polyunsaturated fat. This is also considered a good fat. Sources include fish, flaxseeds, and walnuts. This kind of fat can also be found in seeds and legumes.
4. Trans fat. This is generally considered bad because it could have a negative impact on blood cholesterol. Trans fats are the only man-made kind of fats. Avoid trans fats or consume only minimally.

Vitamins and Minerals

These are substances that are needed by enzymes in our body for energy utilization and growth. Examples of vitamins are vitamins A, B-complex, C, D, E, and K. Examples of minerals are calcium, chromium, and zinc. The best and easiest way to get your vitamins and minerals is by eating a balanced diet. If you are on a vegetarian diet, you need supplementation with B-complex vitamins, especially B12.

Medications:
How They Hurt and Help

Some medications cause weight gain while others can facilitate weight loss. Following are a few examples.

Medications that cause weight gain: The list of medications commonly prescribed in clinical practice that cause obesity is very long. Some of these include:

- Antidepressants
- Antipsychotic medications
- Diabetic drugs
- Beta blockers

- Calcium channel blockers
- Anti-seizure medications
- Steroids
- Antihistamines

If you are on prescription medications and struggling to lose weight, you should talk with your healthcare provider to make sure your medications are not contributing to the weight problem. Many times, a more weight-neutral alternative may be available and appropriate.

Medications that facilitate weight loss: Sometimes diet and exercise are not enough to produce the desired weight loss. You may be a candidate for weight-loss medication if you haven't been able to lose weight through diet and exercise and have one of the following:

- A body mass index (BMI) greater than 30.
- A body mass index (BMI) greater than 27 and obesity-related health problems like diabetes, high cholesterol, arthritis, and high blood pressure.

Weight-loss medications are not a substitute for diet and exercise. They are part of a comprehensive program. When combined with diet and regular exercise, they can result in weight loss of 5 to 10% of total body weight within a year.

Weight-loss medications may not work for everyone.

The following table shows currently available prescription weight-loss medications.

Medication	How it Works	Side Effects	CAUTION
Phentermine			
Has been around for over 55 years Dosing: once a day Approved for short-term use up to 12 weeks. Long-term use is off label	Suppresses appetite Increases feeling of fullness Improves eating behavior and controls cravings May improve energy level	Irritability, insomnia, dry mouth, light headedness, palpitations, constipation, difficulty urinating, headache, tremors.	*Avoid in case of:* Pregnancy Lactation Previous allergy to phentermine Severe heart disease Moderate-severe hypertension Hyperthyroidism Glaucoma Agitated state History of drug abuse *Caution:* SSRI use, other diet medications, primary pulmonary hypertension, valvular heart disease, tolerance, inability to drive or operate machinery.

Diethylproprion (Tenuate)				
Dosing: Once a day Approved for short-term use up to 12 weeks. Long-term use is off label	Similar to phentermine Shorter duration of action	Similar to phentermine Side effects tend to be less severe than in phentermine	Similar to phentermine	
Phendimetrazine				
Dosing: 3 times a day Approved for short-term use up to 12 weeks. Long-term use is off label	Similar to phentermine	Similar to phentermine	Similar to phentermine	
Phentermine/Topiramate (Qsymia)				
Dosing: once a day Approved for long-term use	Decreases appetite Increases feeling of fullness Controls cravings	Pins and needles sensation, headache, dizziness, altered taste, insomnia, constipation, dry mouth. Less frequent: memory loss, nausea, depression, dyslexia	*Avoid in case of:* Pregnancy Lactation Caution Glaucoma Kidney stones	

Medication	How it Works	Side Effects	CAUTION
Contrave Bupropion/Naltrexone combination			
Dosing: once a day Approved for long-term use	Decreases appetite Increases feeling of fullness	Nausea, constipation, headache, vomiting, dizziness, insomnia, dry mouth, diarrhea *Rare side effects:* Suicidal thoughts, mania, seizures, high blood pressure and increase in heart rate. Angle closure glaucoma and severe allergic reaction	*Avoid in case of:* Uncontrolled hypertension Seizure disorder Use of other bupropion containing meds Opioids or opioid antagonist use Pregnancy Lactation Monoamine oxidase inhibitors
Liraglutide (Saxenda)			
Dosing: once a day by injection Approved for long-term use	Slows stomach emptying Increases feeling of fullness	Nausea, vomiting, pancreatitis	Thyroid tumors have been observed in animal studies but not reported in humans

Lorcaserin (Belviq)			
Dosing: twice a day Approved for long-term use	Decreases appetite Increases feeling of fullness	Headache, dizziness, nausea, diarrhea	*Avoid in case of:* Pregnancy
Orlistat			
• Prescription-strength Xenical • OTC-Alli Dosing: 3 times a day Approved for long-term use	Blocks absorption of fat in the intestine	Abdominal discomfort Oily stool and diarrhea Increased flatus	

Other Suggestions for Helping You Lose Weight and Keep It Off

Get support by joining a support group. Such groups provide a safe and educational environment that can inspire success. Studies have shown that dieters who participate in support groups lose more weight than those who do not. Support groups provide a safe place to be yourself. In my experience the groups are very dynamic and have an energy that propels members towards their goals. Within a few weeks, group members become friends. They understand each other's struggles and challenges. They provide motivation and encouragement to each other. They share information and recipes and they celebrate each other's successes.

Elicit the support of family, friends, and community groups such as a church group. Discuss your weight-loss goals with them and ask them to help keep you accountable when you start to stray. Taking weight off and keeping it off requires constant vigilance, and you can use all the help you can get. It is important to realize that not all your friends and family members will be on board with your new lifestyle. You have to be on the lookout for acts of "kindness" that may in fact be counting against your goal and lifestyle. You have to own your decisions.

Use medications. Obesity is now correctly recognized as a disease, and prescription drugs are available to treat it. They help to control appetite and cravings and can increase a sense of fullness. Some of the medications may give you improved energy that will make it easier to move more and to exercise. It is important to note that there are well-known medical problems, such as hormonal problems, sleep apnea, and metabolic syndrome, that make losing weight very difficult. A lot of patients are on medications that hinder weight loss. Commonly used drugs, such as antidepressants and steroids, can also make the hard work of losing weight even harder.

Have surgery. For those with a lot of weight to lose, surgery could be a life-saving measure. It is very effective and it creates the space and time needed to make the lifestyle changes that will lead to lasting success.

Use supplements, including meal replacements and over-the-counter diet pills, but be sure to check with your doctor first. The marketplace is filled with such products, and it can be hard to know which ones to trust. Be aware that the supplement industry, unlike the pharmaceutical industry, is not subject to rigorous standards.

Meal Prep Basics

Preparing your meals in advance can be both fun and empowering. It will give you considerable control over your weight-loss process. Selecting and preparing what you put in your body is so important that it warrants spending time to get it right.

Why Meal Prep?

- Saves money
- Saves time
- Keeps you on track
- Reduces stress
- Reduces mindless eating

Steps

1. Plan your meals and snacks ahead of time.
2. Make a grocery list.
3. Cook your meals, including proteins, vegetables, and carbohydrates.
4. Choose right-size portions.
5. Store.

Supplies

1. Food scale
2. Containers
3. Ziplock bags
4. Cooler
5. Insulated meal bags

How to Make Vegetables More Appealing

A lot of people think that vegetables are boring and monotonous. But if you get creative, you will be amazed by how many ways you can make vegetables tasty and appealing. They can be part of your weight-loss arsenal, your weapon against feeling hungry. If you could make vegetables tasty, you could treat yourself any time you wish. This is because vegetables are essentially free foods. That is, you are not likely to pack extra calories by eating vegetables because your body spends more calories breaking down vegetables than you get from eating them. So why not take the time to learn how to make this important food group work for you? Here are some ways to help you get started:

- Roast or bake to taste. Bake with olive oil.
- Transform with herbs and spices.
- Use dips. Try hummus, low-fat dips, low-fat yogurt.
- Try juicing.
- Mix with fruits in a salad bowl.
- Try veggie rice.
- Swap veggies crisps for chips.
- Stir fry.
- Try vegetable soup.

How to roast vegetables:

1. Preheat oven to 425 degrees.
2. Chop your vegetables.
3. Drizzle lightly with olive oil.
4. Season to taste with herbs, spices, pepper.
5. Spread in a single layer on a baking sheet.
6. Roast until lightly brown.

Get creative, and bon appetit.

Portable Protein

Protein sources can be very useful as snacks or meal replacements. They are a healthy substitute for snacks that are high in sugar and refined carbohydrates. Here is a list of protein sources that are portable and handy:

- Protein shakes are a great way to get the protein you need while limiting the calories and fat that usually accompany typical sources of protein such as meat. Look at the label to make sure the sugar content is not high. I prefer protein shakes with six grams or less of sugar.
- Boiled eggs are high in vitamin B. As snacks, they can keep you full in between meals.
- Roasted chickpeas are nutrient rich and a good source of fiber.
- Edamame are a good source of protein and minerals.
- Yogurt and fruit parfaits—preferably low-fat and with a limited amount of sugar. You may improve palatability by adding spices such as cinnamon or a small amount of a sweetener such as xylitol.
- Cottage cheese is relatively low in calories and high in protein.
- Nuts, such as almonds, pistachios, and macadamia nuts, are calorie dense, so use only a handful.
- Hummus, used as a dip for veggies, can be filling and a healthy snack.
- Low-fat cheese sticks make a handy snack.
- Celery sticks and peanut butter are easy to prepare.

More FIX Menus and Recipes

Breakfast Recipes

Raspberry Gluten-Free Rolled Oatmeal

Ingredients:

1 cup raspberries, fresh or frozen (or any other fruits on hand)
1 cup gluten-free rolled oats
1 tablespoon coconut sugar or xylitol or stevia
1 pinch salt
1 tablespoon coconut oil, olive oil, or macadamia nut oil
4 tablespoon almonds, cashews, pecans, or pistachio pieces
    (optional)
1 cup almond or coconut milk
2 cups water

Directions:

1. Melt oil over medium heat in medium saucepan.
2. Add gluten-free oatmeal to saucepan.
3. Sir occasionally for about 2–3 minutes.
4. Add milk, water, sugar, and salt.
5. Mix well.
6. Bring to a boil.
7. Reduce heat, cover, and simmer for about 20 minutes.
8. Stir occasionally.
9. Turn off heat and let stand for about 5 minutes.
10. Add raspberries (or fruit of choice)
11. Serve 2 tablespoon nuts with each portion (optional)

Easy Overnight Oats
with Chia Seeds

Serves 1
Preparation time: 8 hours
Ready in 10 minutes

Ingredients:

3/4 cup gluten-free rolled oats
1/4 cup almond or coconut milk
1/2 cup water
1 heaping tablespoon chia seeds
1/2–1 tablespoon raw organic honey
1/4 teaspoon cinnamon
Dash of vanilla bean powder or extract
Fruit of choice

Directions:

1. Place oats, liquid, chia seeds, raw organic honey, cinnamon, and vanilla into a 16-ounce mason jar or container of choice. Mix well. Seal shut and place jar in refrigerator overnight.
2. In the morning, mix again and top with anything you'd like, such as fresh fruit, more chia seeds, or cacao nibs.

Simple Scrambled Eggs

Serves 1
(Add any toppings from the FIX List™.)

Ingredients:

2 large eggs
kosher salt and freshly ground black pepper
2 tablespoons unsalted ghee

Directions:

1. Lightly beat the eggs, 3/4 teaspoon salt, and a few grinds of black pepper in a medium bowl.
2. Melt 1 tablespoon of the unsalted ghee in a medium nonstick skillet over low heat; swirl to coat the bottom and sides.
3. Add the eggs, and cook slowly, scraping them up with a rubber spatula occasionally, until most of the liquid has thickened and the eggs are soft, about 10 minutes. (If you like your eggs a little firmer, cook them for an additional 2 to 3 minutes.)
4. Remove them from the heat, and gently fold in the remaining 1 tablespoon of butter. Serve hot.

Vanilla Almond Overnight Oatmeal with Blueberries

Serves 1

Ingredients:

1/2 cup old-fashioned rolled oats
1 cup almond milk, unsweetened original flavor
1 teaspoon honey
1/4 teaspoon pure vanilla extract
sliced, toasted almonds
1/2 cup blueberries

Directions:

1. In a 16-ounce mason jar (or other airtight container that can hold at least 2 cups), combine the oats, almond milk, honey, and vanilla extract. Close with the lid and shake to combine. Refrigerate for 8 hours, or up to 5 days.
2. When ready to eat, heat in the microwave for 2 minutes. Remember to remove the metal lid! Add in desired number of almonds and blueberries.

Vegan Breakfast Bowl

Serves 2

Ingredients:

1 cup gluten-free oats
14 ounces coconut milk
1 cup blueberries
1 cup strawberries
1 cup almonds
1 cup raspberries
1–2 tablespoons nut butter of choice
2 tablespoons coconut flakes
1–2 tablespoons raw organic honey, to taste

Directions:

1. Add the coconut milk and the oats to a saucepan and bring to a boil. Cook for 10 minutes on low heat. Stir in the maple syrup.
2. Wash the berries. Add the oats, berries, and almonds to a bowl. Sprinkle with some coconut flakes and nut butter of your choice.

Israeli Salad

Preparation time: 20 minutes
Serves 4–6

Ingredients:

2 extra-large tomatoes
1 English cucumber
1/2 medium red onion
1 red bell pepper
1 yellow bell pepper
1/2 cup herbs (Italian parsley, mint, or cilantro, or a mix)
zest of one lemon
lemon juice (start with 1/2 a lemon, more to taste)
4 tablespoons olive oil
salt and pepper, to taste

Directions:

1. Chop the first 6 ingredients into a very small fine dice—the smaller, the better.
2. Place in a large bowl and toss with the lemon zest, lemon juice, olive oil, salt, pepper.

Summer Quinoa Salad Bowl

Preparation time: 15 minutes
Makes 1 bowl

Ingredients for the lemon dressing:

1/4 cup olive oil
2 tablespoons fresh lemon juice
2 tablespoons vinegar
1 clove garlic, minced
2 teaspoons honey
pinch of salt and freshly ground black pepper, to taste

Ingredients for the quinoa bowl:

2 cups arugula
1/2 cup cooked quinoa
4 asparagus spears, cooked and cut into 1-inch pieces
1/4 cup peas
2 radishes, sliced
1/2 avocado, sliced
1 hardboiled egg, sliced
2 tablespoons chopped almonds
salt and black pepper, to taste

Directions:

1. In a small bowl or jar, whisk together the olive oil, lemon juice, vinegar, garlic, honey, salt, and pepper. Set aside.
2. Place the arugula in a salad bowl. Top the arugula with the quinoa, asparagus, peas, radishes, avocado, egg slices, and almonds. Drizzle with dressing and season with salt and pepper, to taste. Serve immediately.

Kale and Chicken Caesar Salad

Serves 4
Preparation time: 40 minutes

Ingredients for the salad:

2 bunches of green kale
1 avocado, diced
1/2 cup grated Parmesan cheese

Ingredients for the Caesar dressing:

1 egg (must be room temp!)
1 cup of safflower oil
1/2 teaspoon salt (ideally, kosher)
2 teaspoons Dijon mustard
juice of 1 lemon
6–8 flat anchovy filets in olive oil
4 cloves garlic
2 tablespoon red wine vinegar

Ingredients for the chicken:

6 boneless, skinless chicken breasts
2 tablespoons olive oil
2 tablespoons lemon juice
1 teaspoon garlic powder, or to taste
kosher salt, to taste
black pepper, to taste

Directions:

1. In a bowl or ziplock bag, combine all of the "for the chicken"
   ingredients together and toss so that the chicken is coated evenly.
   Set aside and allow to marinade for 15–30 minutes, at room
   temperature.

2. Preheat oven to 400 degrees.
3. Meanwhile, make the Caesar dressing: If your egg is chilled, place it in a cup of hot or very warm water for 3–5 minutes to bring it to room temp. *Your egg must be at room temperature or your dressing will not emulsify.*
4. Place room temperature egg, the kosher salt, and 1/4 cup of safflower oil in a food processor or blender, and blend well.
5. Turn your food processor or blender on and keep blending as you *very slowly* pour in the remaining 3/4 cup of safflower oil. After about 3 minutes, you will have a mayo-like consistency.
6. Now, toss the anchovies, garlic, lemon juice, Dijon mustard, and red wine vinegar in with the mayo. Blend until smooth. Taste, and add more salt and pepper to taste. Add more anchovies or red wine vinegar if you wish. Set the dressing aside while you prepare your salad.
7. Rinse and pat dry the kale. Remove kale from the stem, then chop it up so that it is diced very small. Place the chopped kale in a large bowl and set aside.
8. Heat a cast iron skillet or an oven safe skillet over medium-high heat. When skillet is hot, place chicken breasts in skillet and sear on both sides until they are lightly browned, about 3–4 minutes per side.
9. Place the skillet into the preheated oven and let the chicken continue to cook all the way through in the oven. Depending on the thickness of the chicken, it should take between 10 and 15 minutes.
10. While the chicken is cooking, pour desired amount of the Caesar salad dressing over the chopped kale, toss to coat evenly, and set aside to let the kale marinate in the dressing—this allows the kale to soften a bit so that it doesn't have too much of a bite to it.
11. Remove chicken from the oven and, using tongs, transfer onto a cutting board. Let it rest on the cutting board for about 5 minutes to allow juices to settle back into the chicken.

Spinach Salad with Chicken, Eggs, and Avocado

Serves 1

Ingredients:

3 cups fresh spinach, torn, stems removed
2 boiled eggs, sliced
3 ounces chopped precooked chicken
1 ripe avocado, diced
salt and pepper to taste
1/8 cup of diced red onion (optional)

Directions:

1. Add all ingredients to a large salad bowl.
2. Toss to combine.
3. Top with seasoned chicken.

Roasted Veggie Chickpea Salad

Serves 6–8

Ingredients:

3 bunches arugula leaves or mixed greens
2 1/2 cups butternut squash, peeled and diced
5 peeled and precooked beets (or roast the beets yourself), chopped
1 (15-ounce) can chickpeas, rinsed and drained
1 pint cherry or plum tomatoes, halved
1/3 cup extra-virgin olive oil, plus 2 tablespoons
1/4 cup freshly squeezed orange juice
kosher salt and freshly ground pepper, to taste

Directions:

1. Preheat oven to 400 degrees.
2. Toss cubed butternut squash with 2 tablespoons olive oil and season generously with salt and pepper.
3. Spread out on a baking sheet in an even layer and bake for 45–50 minutes, or until fork tender.
4. Transfer butternut squash to a large serving bowl and add chopped beets, arugula, and halved tomatoes. Add in chickpeas.
5. In a small bowl or glass, whisk together olive oil and orange juice until combined.
6. Drizzle salad dressing over peas and vegetables and gently toss together until everything is coated.
7. Taste and adjust seasoning, if necessary, and serve immediately. Note: if roasting beets at home, place beets in a baking dish with 1/2 cup water. Cover with aluminum foil and bake at 400 degrees for 50–60 minutes, or until fork tender. Let cool before peeling.

Simple Summer Zucchini and Tomato "Pasta" (or use gluten-free pasta)

Yield: 4 servings
Preparation time: 5 minutes
Cook time: 5–10 minutes

Ingredients:

1 green zucchini
1 yellow zucchini
1 clove garlic, crushed
1/2 cup packed fresh parsley, rinsed and dried
2 tablespoons butter or ghee (substitute coconut oil for dairy free)
sea salt and pepper to taste
1 cup chopped baby tomatoes

Directions:

1. Make zucchinis into noodles with a spiralizer or julienne peeler (can be bought readily).
2. Place a large frying pan on the stove on medium heat.
3. Add the ghee or coconut butter, parsley, and garlic to the pan and sauté for a few minutes.
4. Add the zucchini noodles to the pan and sauté for another 5 or so minutes until the noodles have the desired texture.
5. Add salt and pepper and mix well.
6. Remove from heat and add chopped baby tomatoes. Toss to combine.
7. Serve and enjoy!

Honey-Dijon Chicken, Roasted Carrots, and Roasted Sweet Potato

Ingredients for the chicken:

2 tablespoons honey
2 tablespoons Dijon mustard
1 tablespoon extra-virgin olive oil, plus more for grill
1/2 teaspoon kosher salt
freshly ground black pepper
4 boneless, skinless chicken breasts, butterflied
1 lime, cut into wedges

Ingredients for the roasted carrots:

12 carrots
3 tablespoons good olive oil
1 1/4 teaspoons kosher salt
1/2 teaspoon freshly ground black pepper
2 tablespoons minced fresh dill or parsley

Directions:

1. Preheat oven to 400 degrees.
2. If the carrots are thick, cut them in half lengthwise; if not, leave whole. Slice the carrots diagonally in 1 1/2-inch-thick slices. (The carrots will shrink while cooking so make the slices big.)
3. Toss them in a bowl with the olive oil, salt, and pepper. Transfer to a sheet pan in 1 layer and roast in the oven for 20 minutes, until browned and tender.
4. Toss the carrots with minced dill or parsley, season to taste, and serve.

Ingredients for the roasted sweet potato:

1 large sweet potato
2 tablespoons olive oil
1 tablespoon garlic powder
1/4 teaspoon sea salt
1/8 teaspoon pepper

Directions:

1. Preheat oven to 400 degrees.
2. Cut off ends of sweet potato.
3. Once sliced, toss in bowl and drizzle olive oil with salt, pepper, and garlic powder.
4. Roast in oven for 20–25 minutes.

Mexican Zucchini Beef Skillet

Ingredients:

1 1/2 medium zucchinis, sliced and quartered
1 pound ground beef
1 1/2 cloves garlic minced
4 1/2 cups salsa
3/4 tablespoon chili powder
3/4 teaspoon ground cumin
3/4 teaspoon salt
3/4 teaspoon black pepper
1/4 teaspoon onion powder
1/4 teaspoon crushed red pepper flakes

Directions:

1. Brown ground beef with minced garlic, salt, and pepper.
2. Cook over medium heat until meat is browned.
3. Add tomatoes and remaining spices. Cover and simmer on low heat for another 10 minutes.
4. Add the zucchini. Cover and cook for about 10 more minutes until zucchini is cooked, but still firm.

Zucchini Spirals with Red Sauce

Yield: 4 servings
Total time: 30 minutes
Preparation time: 10 minutes

Ingredients:

2 tablespoons extra virgin olive oil
1/2 cup diced white onions
6 garlic cloves, peeled and minced (or pressed)
1 (28-ounce) can diced tomatoes
2 tablespoons tomato paste
1/2 cup roughly-chopped fresh basil leaves, loosely packed
1 1/2 teaspoons coarse salt
1/4 teaspoon black pepper
1/8 teaspoon crushed red pepper flakes (or a pinch of cayenne)
2 large zucchinis, spiralized
freshly-grated Parmesan cheese, for grating

Directions:

1. Heat oil in a large sauté pan over medium-high heat.
2. Add onions and sauté for 5 minutes, stirring occasionally, until the onions are soft and translucent.
3. Add garlic and sauté for 1 minute, stirring frequently, until fragrant.
4. Add in the tomatoes, tomato paste, basil, salt, pepper, and crushed red pepper flakes, then stir to combine. Continue cooking until the sauce reaches a simmer.
5. Reduce heat to medium-low and continue to let the sauce simmer for about 15 minutes, or until the oil on the surface is a deep orange and the sauce is reduced and thickened. Taste, and season the sauce with additional salt and pepper if needed.

6. Add in the spiralized zucchini and toss until it is evenly coated with sauce. Continue to cook for 2–3 minutes until the noodles are slightly softened.
7. Remove from the heat and serve immediately, garnished with Parmesan cheese.

Garlic and Rosemary Grilled Lamb Chops

Serves 4 people

Ingredients:

2 pounds lamb loin or rib chops (thick cut)
4 cloves garlic, minced
1 tablespoon fresh rosemary, chopped
1 1/4 teaspoon kosher salt
1/2 teaspoon ground black pepper
zest of 1 lemon
1/4 cup olive oil

Directions:

1. Combine the garlic, rosemary, salt, pepper, lemon zest, and olive oil in a measuring cup.
2. Pour the marinade over the lamb chops, making sure to flip them over to cover them completely. Cover and marinate the chops in the fridge for as little as 1 hour, or as long as overnight.
3. Heat your grill to medium-high heat, then sear the lamb chops for 2–3 minutes, on each side. Lower the heat to medium then cook them for 5–6 minutes, or until the internal temperature reads 150 degrees.
4. Allow the lamb chops to rest on a plate covered with aluminum foil for 5 minutes before serving.

Grass-Fed Beef Burger Bowls

Yield: 2 servings
Preparation time: 10 minutes
Cooking time: 20 minutes

Ingredients:

8 ounces ground beef
1 onion, sliced
4 cups spinach
1 lemon, juiced
1 tablespoon olive oil
1 tomato, sliced
1 medium sweet tomato, peeled, sliced, and roasted
salt and pepper

Directions:

1. Form the ground beef into two equal-sized 4-ounce patties and season with salt and pepper. Make an indentation in the center of the patty. Place on a hot grill or skillet. Cook for 4–5 minutes on each side, or until it is cooked to the desired temperature.
2. Also place onion slices on grill or skillet to caramelize. Cook for 2–3 minutes on each side.
3. Portion out the romaine into two bowls. Mix together the lemon juice and olive oil, and dress the lettuce. Top with the tomato slices, sweet potato, and onion.
4. Let burger patty cool for 5 minutes, then place on top of the burger bowl.
5. Add ketchup, mustard, or other condiments as desired.

Vegan Pesto or Tomato Sauce Spaghetti Squash

Serves 2

Ingredients:

1 medium spaghetti squash
1 cup packed kale
1/2 cup packed basil leaves
1/2 cup walnuts
1/2 cup olive oil
2 cloves garlic
1/4 teaspoon salt, or more to taste

Directions:

1. Place spaghetti squash cut side down in a baking dish. Add about 1 inch of water. Poke 6 slits through the skin of each squash half. Microwave for about 12–15 minutes or until tender.
2. For the pesto, combine all the ingredients (kale through salt) in a mini food processor. Blend together until pureed.
3. Top spaghetti squash with desired amount of pesto.
4. Season to taste with salt and pepper.

Mexican Stuffed Peppers

Serves 4

Ingredients:

4 large bell peppers
3/4 cup dry quinoa
15 ounce can black beans
1 cup corn
2 green onions
2/3 cup salsa
2 tablespoons nutritional yeast
1 1/2 teaspoon cumin
1 teaspoon smoked paprika
1 teaspoon chili powder

Directions:

1. Preheat oven to 350.
2. Cook quinoa according to package directions with 1 1/2 cups water/broth.
3. While quinoa is cooking, halve bell peppers and remove stems, seeds and ribs.
4. Rinse and drain black beans, thaw corn, and slice green onions.
5. In a large mixing bowl, add cooked quinoa and all other ingredients except bell peppers. Stir to combine, and adjust taste if needed.
6. In a lightly sprayed 9 x 13-inch baking dish, place pepper halves, and generously stuff them with the quinoa filling. Lightly press down to compact and fill all the crevices.
7. Cover with tin foil and bake for 35–40 minutes. Remove foil, and bake 10 minutes more.

Notes:

_____

_____

_____

_____

_____

_____

_____

_____

_____

_____

_____

_____

_____

_____

_____

_____

_____

_____

_____

_____

_____

_____

_____

_____

_____

_____

_____

_____

Notes:

_____

_____

_____

_____

_____

_____

_____

_____

_____

_____

_____

_____

_____

_____

_____

_____

_____

_____

_____

_____

_____

_____

_____

_____

_____

_____

_____

_____

References

1. National Institute of Diabetes and Digestive and Kidney Diseases, "Overweight & Obesity Statistics," https://www.niddk.nih.gov/health-information/health-statistics/overweight-obesity.

2. Harriet Brown, "The Weight of the Evidence," *Slate*, March 24, 2015, www.slate.com.

3. Sara Police, "How Much Have Obesity Rates Risen Since 1950? LIVESTRONG.COM, https://www.livestrong.com/article/384722-how-much-have-obesity-rates-risen-since-1950/.

4. D. B. Allison, et al., "Annual deaths attributable to obesity in the United States," *JAMA* 282, no. 16 (October 1999): 1530–1538.

5. J. E. Manson, et al., "Body Weight and Mortality among Women," *New England Journal of Medicine* 333, no. 11 (1995): 677–685.

6. G. Whitlock, et al., "Body-mass Index and Cause-specific Mortality in 900,000 Adults: Collaborative Analyses of 57 Prospective Studies," *Lancet* 373, no. 9669 (March 2009): 1083–1096.

7. Anne B. Newman, MD, MPH, et al., "Association of Long-Distance Corridor Walk Performance with Mortality, Cardiovascular Disease, Mobility Limitation, and Disability," *JAMA* 295, no. 17 (2006): 2018–2026. doi: 10.1001/jama.295.17.2018

8. A. F. Dor, C. Langwith, and E. Tan. "A Heavy Burden: The Individual Costs of Being Overweight and Obese in the United States," George Washington University of Public Health and Health Services Department of Health Policy, 2010, http://hsrc.himmelfarb.gwu.edu/sphhs_policy_facpubs/212/.

9. Giueseppe Passarino, Francesco De Rango, and Alberto Montesanto, "Human Longevity: Genetics or Lifestyle? It Takes Two to Tango," *Immunity & Ageing* 13 (2016):12.

10. Life Expectancy in the USA, 1900–98. U.demog.berkeley.edu ~andrew/1918/figure2.html.

11. Bloomburg School of Public Health, Johns Hopkins, "Study Suggests 86 Percent of Americans Could be Overweight or Obese by 2030" (July 29, 2008), https://www.jhsph.edu/news/news-releases /2008/wang-obesity-projections.html.

12. ABC News Staff, "100 Million Dieters, $20 Billion: The Weight-Loss Industry by the Numbers" (May 18, 2012), http://abcnews.go .com/Health/100-million-dieters-20-billion-weight-loss-industry /story?id=16297197.

13. Mathew Boesler, "CHART OF THE DAY: The Moment When American Calorie Consumption Went Ballistic," *Business Insider*, http://www.businessinsider.com/us-calorie-consumption-surged-in -the-80s-2013-9.

14. Alice G. Walton, "How Much Sugar Are Americans Eating?" [Infographic], *Forbes* (2012), https://www.forbes.com/sites/alicegwal ton/2012/08/30/how-much-sugar-are-americans-eating-infographic /#1ab03cad4ee7.

15. G. Vighi et al. "Allergy and the Gastrointestinal System," *Clinical and Experimental Immunology* 153, Suppl 1 (2008): 3–6, https:// www.ncbi.nlm.nih.gov/pubmed/?term=Vighi%20G%5BAuthor%5D &cauthor=true&cauthor_uid=18721321.

16. Jessica Stoller-Conrad, "Microbes Help Produce Serotonin in Gut," Caltech, www.caltech.edu/news/microbes-help-produce -serotonin-gut-46495.

17. Jessica Hamzelou, "Boost C-section Babies by Giving Them Vaginal Bacteria," *New Scientist*, https://www.newscientist.com/article /2075768-boost-c-section-babies-by-giving-them-vaginal-bacteria/.

18. National Center for Health Statistics, "Exercise or Physical Activity," https://www.cdc.gov/nchs/fastats/exercise.htm.